# MICROCOMPUTERS and PHYSIOLOGICAL SIMULATION

# MICROCOMPUTERS and PHYSIOLOGICAL SIMULATION

## James E. Randall

*Indiana University*
*School of Medicine*
*Bloomington, Indiana*

Foreword by

## Arthur C. Guyton

*University of Mississippi*
*School of Medicine*
*Jackson, Mississippi*

1980

Addison-Wesley Publishing Company, Inc.
Advanced Book Program
Reading, Massachusetts

London · Amsterdam · Don Mills, Ontario · Sydney · Tokyo

**Library of Congress Cataloging in Publication Data**

Randall, James Edwin.
  Microcomputers and physiological simulation.

  Includes bibliographical references and index.
  1. Physiology—Data processing.  2. Physiology—
Mathematical models.  3. Physiology—Study and teaching—
Simulation methods.  4. Microcomputers.
  I. Title.  [DNLM:  1. Computers.  2. Physiology.
3. Models, Biological.   QT26.5 R188m]
QP33.6.D38R36        599.01'028'54        79-27675
ISBN 0-201-06128-7

Reproduced by Addison-Wesley Publishing Company, Inc., Advanced Book Program, Reading, Massachusetts, from camera-ready copy prepared at the office of the author.

Copyright © 1980 by Addison-Wesley Publishing Company, Inc.
Published simultaneously in Canada.

Manufactured in the United States of America

ABCDEFGHIJ-AL-89876543210

CONTENTS

FOREWORD by ARTHUR C. GUYTON . . . . . . . . . . . . . . . . ix

PREFACE . . . . . . . . . . . . . . . . . . . . . . . . . . xiii

1.  INTRODUCTION . . . . . . . . . . . . . . . . . . . .   1

        Mechanical Models . . . . . . . . . . . . . . . . .   2
        Mathematical Models. . . . . . . . . . . . . . . . .   3
        Analog Computers . . . . . . . . . . . . . . . . . .   4
        Digital Computers. . . . . . . . . . . . . . . . . .   5
        Teaching by Simulation . . . . . . . . . . . . . . .   7
        References . . . . . . . . . . . . . . . . . . . . .   8


2.  MICROCOMPUTER COMPONENTS. . . . . . . . . . . . . . .   9

        Microprocessors . . . . . . . . . . . . . . . . . .  11
        Semiconductor Memory . . . . . . . . . . . . . . . .  14
        Keyboard . . . . . . . . . . . . . . . . . . . . . .  16
        Cathode Ray Tube Displays . . . . . . . . . . . . .  17
        Mass Storage . . . . . . . . . . . . . . . . . . . .  20
        Microcomputers . . . . . . . . . . . . . . . . . . .  24
        References . . . . . . . . . . . . . . . . . . . . .  26
        Microcomputer Periodicals. . . . . . . . . . . . . .  27
        Manufacturers Cited . . . . . . . . . . . . . . . .  27


3.  OPERATING SYSTEMS AND PROGRAMMING LANGUAGES . . . . . .  29

        Monitors and Operating Systems . . . . . . . . . . .  30
        CP/M . . . . . . . . . . . . . . . . . . . . . . . .  32
        Assemblers . . . . . . . . . . . . . . . . . . . . .  34
        BASIC . . . . . . . . . . . . . . . . . . . . . . .  35
        Other Programming Languages. . . . . . . . . . . . .  37
        References . . . . . . . . . . . . . . . . . . . . .  38
        Software Sources . . . . . . . . . . . . . . . . . .  38

4.  HARDWARE ENHANCEMENTS FOR SIMULATION . . . . . . . . .    39

        Graphics . . . . . . . . . . . . . . . . . . . . .    40
        Numerical Processors . . . . . . . . . . . . . . .    44
        References . . . . . . . . . . . . . . . . . . . .    49
        Manufacturers Cited. . . . . . . . . . . . . . . .    49


5.  REPRESENTATIVE MICROCOMPUTERS . . . . . . . . . . . . .    50

        TRS-80 . . . . . . . . . . . . . . . . . . . . . .    51
        Apple II . . . . . . . . . . . . . . . . . . . . .    52
        S-100 Bus Microcomputer. . . . . . . . . . . . . .    55
        References . . . . . . . . . . . . . . . . . . . .    56


6.  COMPARTMENTAL KINETICS: A FIRST EXAMPLE . . . . . . . .    57

        The Hydraulic Model. . . . . . . . . . . . . . . .    58
        Computed Responses . . . . . . . . . . . . . . . .    59
        The BASIC Program  . . . . . . . . . . . . . . . .    61
        References . . . . . . . . . . . . . . . . . . . .    64
        Chapter Appendix . . . . . . . . . . . . . . . . .    64

7.  THE GLUCOSE TOLERANCE TEST. . . . . . . . . . . . . . .    69

        The Insulin-Glucose Interaction Model. . . . . . .    70
        The BASIC Program. . . . . . . . . . . . . . . . .    73
        Computed Responses . . . . . . . . . . . . . . . .    76
        References . . . . . . . . . . . . . . . . . . . .    79
        Chapter Appendix . . . . . . . . . . . . . . . . .    79


8.  CARDIOVASCULAR SYSTEM MECHANICS . . . . . . . . . . . .    83

        The Functional Relationships . . . . . . . . . . .    85
        Steady-State Solutions . . . . . . . . . . . . . .    91
        Steady-State Exercises . . . . . . . . . . . . . .   101
        Transient Solutions. . . . . . . . . . . . . . . .   105
        References . . . . . . . . . . . . . . . . . . . .   112
        Chapter Appendix . . . . . . . . . . . . . . . . .   112


9.  ARTERIAL PULSE PRESSURE . . . . . . . . . . . . . . . .   116

        The Model  . . . . . . . . . . . . . . . . . . . .   116
        Computed Responses . . . . . . . . . . . . . . . .   118
        The BASIC Program  . . . . . . . . . . . . . . . .   121
        References . . . . . . . . . . . . . . . . . . . .   126
        Chapter Appendix . . . . . . . . . . . . . . . . .   126

10. VECTORCARDIOGRAPHY AND THE LIMB LEADS . . . . . . . . . .   129

        Computed Responses . . . . . . . . . . . . . . . . .   131
        The BASIC Program  . . . . . . . . . . . . . . . . .   133
        Chapter Appendix . . . . . . . . . . . . . . . . . .   137


11. DISTORTION OF WAVEFORMS . . . . . . . . . . . . . . . . .   140

        Computed Responses . . . . . . . . . . . . . . . . .   141
        Digital Filtering  . . . . . . . . . . . . . . . . .   145
        Restoring Distorted Waveforms  . . . . . . . . . . .   147
        The BASIC Program  . . . . . . . . . . . . . . . . .   150
        References . . . . . . . . . . . . . . . . . . . . .   152
        Chapter Appendix . . . . . . . . . . . . . . . . . .   152


12. AXON ACTION POTENTIALS  . . . . . . . . . . . . . . . . .   157

        Formulation in BASIC . . . . . . . . . . . . . . . .   159
        Output Displays  . . . . . . . . . . . . . . . . . .   170
        Properties of Excitation . . . . . . . . . . . . . .   177
        Computation Methods  . . . . . . . . . . . . . . . .   187
        References . . . . . . . . . . . . . . . . . . . . .   195
        Chapter Appendix . . . . . . . . . . . . . . . . . .   195

13. CARDIAC ACTION POTENTIALS . . . . . . . . . . . . . . . .   199

        Formulation in BASIC . . . . . . . . . . . . . . . .   201
        Computed Responses . . . . . . . . . . . . . . . . .   208
        Output Display and Computation Methods . . . . . . .   215
        References . . . . . . . . . . . . . . . . . . . . .   221
        Chapter Appendix . . . . . . . . . . . . . . . . . .   221

14. FORMATTING STUDENT EXERCISES  . . . . . . . . . . . . . .   225

        Turnkey Systems  . . . . . . . . . . . . . . . . . .   226
        Programming  . . . . . . . . . . . . . . . . . . . .   228


INDEX . . . . . . . . . . . . . . . . . . . . . . . . . . . .   232

FOREWORD

Though many of us have experienced the effectiveness of
physiological computer simulations as a teaching tool for a
number of years, we have also known that its major limitation
has been cost. For this reason, physiological simulation has
remained the property of research laboratories or of highly
subsidized teaching programs. But, with the coming of the
microcomputer, an order of magnitude decrease in cost has been
achieved so that this should no longer be a limitation.

Fortunately, a few physiologists have been very quick to
recognize the potential of the microcomputer for teaching and
have surged forward to develop the necessary teaching
methodology. So far as I am aware, this book by Dr. James
Randall, Microcomputers and Physiological Simulation, is by far
the most complete effort so far.

In this book, Dr. Randall has approached not only the
theoretical aspects of microcomputing, but also many of the
pragmatic details that answer the question, "How do I get
started?" He has addressed both theory and other information
about the hardware itself that will be valuable not only to the
beginner in this field, but also to those who already have been
long engaged in physiological simulation.

Equally as important, however, are the physiological
exercises that Dr. Randall has outlined in this text. He has
been very forthright in stating that he hopes these are only
forerunners of a multitude of simulations being developed by
many physiologists throughout the world which will be shared
among all for teaching purposes.

These physiologists who have practiced computer
simulaton of physiological mechanisms, without exception, do not
have to be sold on its importance. Yet, it is difficult to
portray to the uninitiated the satisfaction that comes from
fitting together the basic pieces of a physiological mechanism,
and then making the total system function as an integral unit.
It is hard to tell the non-believer that many of the simplest
mechanisms that we have taught for years do not in reality
function exactly as our intuitions have led us to believe. Yet,

when one sees the computer solutions of function, under both
normal and abnormal conditions, one is often lead into new
logical dimensions and certainly to a fuller understanding of
the basic physiology.

    To give a simple example of how our intuition often
fools us, it is very easy to demonstrate, using computer
simulation of basic circulatory hemodynamics, that an increase
in total peripheral resistance can either <u>increase</u> or <u>decrease</u>
the arterial pressure. But how many people have every thought
of increased total peripheral resistance decreasing the
pressure? The hemodynamic answer to this is very simple: when
the increase in total preripheral resistance results from
increased venous resistance, the arterial pressure falls rather
than rises because the increased resistance then decreases
cardiac output far more than it increases the total peripheral
resistance. As simple as this is, almost without exception,
medical students throughout the world are taught that arterial
pressure is mainly controlled by changes in total peripheral
resistance. If we will give heed to that which we can learn
from physiological simulation, we will quickly forget the
relationship between total peripheral resistance and arterial
pressure but will instead speak only of the relationship between
arterial pressure and arterial resistance. This will also allow
us to understand readily why the arterial pressure is not
changed at all by most clinical conditions in which the total
peripheral resistance changes. Such conditions as A-V fistulae,
anemia, thyrotoxicosis, hypothyroidism, and even the loss of all
four limbs can alter the total peripheral resistance through
ranges of several hundred percent.

    Almost certainly, the physiological simulations that are
yet to come will be equally as exciting as those already
accomplished, including simulations of such phenomena as
response of the neuronal cell body to excitatory, facilitatory,
and inhibitory signals; operation of delay line circuits in the
cerebellum for feedback control of motor activity; automatic
gain control in the nervous pathways; contrast control by the
lateral inhibition mechanisms; and many others. In both the
respiratory and circulatory fields many computer models are
already available, but these need to be reduced to teaching
tools, especially to demonstrate to the student the effects of
clinical abnormalities on the overall function of the system.
There is no better way to understand the different causes of
respiratory distress, ranging from emphysema to pneumonia to
ambient hypoxia. And, thus far, no better way has been found to
demonstrate the relationship of kidney abnormalities to the
pathophysiologic results -- edema, hypertension, uremia, and so
forth.

    One can observe that I am a devotee of computer
simulaton of physiological mechanisms, mainly because my own

experience with this technique has been one of the most important learning episodes of my life. It is for this reason that I am delighted to have this opportunity of writing a Foreword for Dr. Randall's book, <u>Microcomputers</u> <u>and</u> <u>Physiological</u> <u>Simulation.</u> Dr. Randall's unique background has made it possible for him to put together this book. His training, especially in the multiple disciplines that are required -- basic physiology, mathematics, computer technology, biophysics, physics, and even complex electronic circuitry -- is reflected in this volume. The development of physiological simulation as a teaching tool is an important type of research in itself that does not come either easily or rapidly. Instead, it requires a high level of personal devotion to teaching and a special commitment to the task itself. I am especially delighted that Dr. Randall has had the interest and drive that has led to this completed task.

Arthur C. Guyton, M. D.

PREFACE

The objective of this book is to further the cause of quantitative physiology by demonstrating to nonspecialists that they can use the new microcomputers for mathematical modeling. The technology which has made the pocket calculator a personal possession is providing microprocessor-based computers at a reasonable cost, even to be purchased in neighborhood shopping centers. These provide considerable computational power and when combined with modern mass storage devices offer significant benefits to individual scientists for record keeping and manuscript writing as well. The accessibility of this hardware, combined with the programming simplicity of BASIC, may mark the beginning of an era in which computers are widely used for formulating and testing biological concepts. The particular approach of this book is to illustrate that microcomputers can provide graphic displays of physiological responses to a wide range of disturbances thereby providing an opportunity for gaining insight regarding the underlying mechanisms of interrelated dynamic processes.

When microcomputers were introduced in 1975 they were in the form of kits which required considerable technical skill to assemble and operate. After an explosive growth period, during which many pioneering manufacturers failed financially, there now appears to be a stable source of assembled microcomputers which are effective in scientific applications. This book addresses representative models requiring three different levels of financial and time commitment.

The TRS-80, available through Radio Shack retail outlets, is attractive as a personal investment because of its powerful BASIC in a compact keyboard unit at a modest initial cost. This model can be used to provide tabular solutions or low-resolution graphic displays of mathematical formulations. The Apple II is suitable for student applications and for the casual programmer who wants reasonable graphics resolution and computation speed in a standardized and integrated configuration conducive for software exchange among different institutions. This is a "turnkey" model which automatically loads and starts the first program from the magnetic disk when the power switch is turned on. It has vector graphics and simple disk operating commands integrated into BASIC. In addition, it can be

conveniently expanded to include a floating point processor   for
the increased speed required for some iterative simulations.

     The serious user may prefer a microcomputer   based   upon
the  S-100 bus, a method of standardizing the interconnection of
components   from   a   variety   of   manufacturers.     CP/M is   a
disk-based    operating    system   which   permits   given   software
(programs)   to   be   run   on   a   variety   of   different   hardware
configurations.    The   use   of   these   standardization   methods
provides maximum computing power for a   variety   of   programming
languages   but their initiation and use does require more than a
casual   commitment.    Their   diversity   is   a   benefit   to   the
individual   installation   but   also   discourages the exchange of
programs because of the variety of options encountered.

     During   the   last   four   years   I have evaluated each of
these microcomputer alternatives as they came upon the market by
using   them   for   teaching demonstrations and student self-study
exercises in medical and graduate physiology courses.    When   I
presented   microcomputer   demonstrations of teaching simulations
at the Learning Resource Center   at   national   meetings   of   the
American   Physiological   Society   it   became   obvious that other
physiologists were very much interested but uncertain about   how
to   implement   the   technique at their own institutions.   It was
within   this   setting   that   the   approach   of   this   book   was
formulated.

     The   first   five   chapters   discuss   the   hardware   and
software   alternatives   for   the person who wishes to purchase a
microcomputer   system.    The   balance   of   the   book   documents
simulations   of increasing complexity as I have used them.   Each
of these chapters presents a commonly   encountered   model   of   a
physiological   process   or   system   and   describes how it can be
implemented in BASIC.    Although   FORTRAN   is   a   more   powerful
language,   perhaps   to   be   replaced by Pascal, BASIC is the one
language available with all microcomputers.    In   spite   of   the
slowness   of   BASIC   its   simplicity   and   familiarity seem more
appropriate than the alternatives for   the   objectives   of   this
introductory   book.    For   similar   reasons   the   differential
equations are solved by simple   rectangular   Euler   integration.
The   BASIC   programs are laid out in modular form for discussion
convenience   and   so   that   the   input/output   routines   may   be
modified    to    suit    the    characteristics   of   the   different
microcomputers.   The chapters conclude with detailed listings of
programs printed directly from the Apple II.

     Chapter 12, which   presents   the   familiar   Hodgkin   and
Huxley   model   for   axon   action potential, may be of particular
interest to people teaching the basics of   neurophysiology.     I
have   found   lecture   demonstrations   of   the   computed membrane
potential and membrane   conductance   changes   to   be   especially
well-received.    In   addition,   the microcomputer   is   used   for

self-study by the students permitting them to explore the
mechanisms of summation, threshold, and accommodation in terms
of the conductance changes in a manner not possible in the
laboratory. Computer simulation can not replace the laboratory
experiment but it certainly does provide unique opportunities
for gaining insight into the mechanisms of dynamic processes.
Even the process of formulating conceptualizations into
programming statements can be a vehicle for learning for both
the instructor and the serious student of physiololology.

I wish to acknowledge the people and the events which
made it possible to produce this volume within a short period of
time. Special credit goes to my Publisher. Her grasp of the
timeliness of the subject matter and the decision to produce it
from camera-ready copy contributed significantly to my diligence
in carrying the project through to its completion. The
procedure for composing and editing the manuscript is typical of
that to be expected as word processors become academic tools.
Text was entered from the keyboard of a microcomputer and viewed
on a video monitor. Individual 5,000-word segments were saved
on a total of five flexible (floppy) diskettes from which any
section could be recalled for editing and for printing pages
with justified margins. The final copy was produced on an
impact printer and combined with positive photographs of the
simulations as they appeared on the video screen. Dr. Barbara
Randall was extremely helpful with her tireless effort to polish
my grammar and provide clarity of presentation. Special
recognition is due to the Indiana Attorney General's Trust Fund,
Microprocessor Project which purchased the SOL microcomputer in
1977, a step that later proved to be critical in the final
production of a professional simulation package.

When first introduced personal computers were promoted
largely on the basis of their capacity for entertainment and
games. One purpose of this volume is to show that they also
have serious scientific applications. The examples happen to
reflect my own personal interests and teaching experience, but
the intent is to stimulate others to take advantage of these new
facilities. Though the hardware costs are reasonable one should
not underestimate the cost in hours of effort involved in
developing software tailored for specific applications. It is
for this reason that I have a strong hope that as others develop
their own teaching exercises that there will be some mechanism
to share these efforts with other institutions.

James E. Randall, Ph. D.

# MICROCOMPUTERS and PHYSIOLOGICAL SIMULATION

Chapter 1

INTRODUCTION

One of the attributes of physiology as a discipline is
that it challenges the abilities of scientists with diverse
backgrounds and interests. Biochemists, pharmacologists,
immunologists, and molecular biologists, to name a few, find
opportunities to bring their own special talents to bear upon
the fundamental processes which are the bases for the function
of living systems. During the last quarter century we have seen
the development of professional biophysicists, bioengineers, and
biomathematicians. Their special approaches to physiological
phenomena frequently emphasize quantitative rigor using
mathematical models implemented on institutional computers.
Unfortunately, this situation tends to create the impression
that mathematical models and simulation are useful only to the
specialists involved.

The recent introduction of microcomputers inexpensive
enough to become personal possessions can place the tools of
applied mathematics in the hands of any physiologist. The
simplicity of programming in BASIC, the conveniences of
ownership, and the computing power offered by modern memory and
mass storage technology now offer new opportunities for
mathematical experimentation by the nonspecialist. The
organization of this book stresses the use of microcomputers for
teaching simulations, but the intent is to introduce applied
mathematics in a form which is palpable to many physiologists.

---

James E. Randall, Microcomputers and Physiological Simulation

Dr. C. J. Dickinson (1977), in his recent book <u>A</u> <u>Computer</u> <u>Model</u> <u>of</u> <u>Human</u> <u>Respiration</u>, eloquently discusses the philosophical aspects of using computer models for teaching physiology. His opening chapter stresses that computers often can solve problems by tireless brute-force for people who may lack mathematical skill or even native intelligence. That book documents a holistic model for human respiration, attempting to simulate the clinical conditions encountered by practicing physicians. The present book tackles smaller segments, the basic concepts encountered by students during their first year of physiology. The material is only a modest beginning toward what can ultimately be achieved by simulating the dynamic interactions between the many variables within the body.

## MECHANICAL MODELS

It is common practice to use mechanical models to illustrate the essential features of physical processes operating within the body. The simpler the model is the stronger the teaching impact. No one seems particularly disturbed by the simplifying assumptions. Examples include the balloon in a bell jar for pulmonary mechanics and the squeeze bulb pumping fluids into an elastic tube analogous to the aorta. A pair of leaky tanks are commonly used to illustrate the washout curves of sequential body compartments.

There have been a number of mechanical cardiovascular models which include components with adjustable parameters, such as pumping rate, peripheral resistance, arterial and venous compliances, total fluid volume, and even a pressure regulator. Using such a model the student gains insight into the fact that the distribution of blood volume, vascular pressures, and flows all depend upon the prevailing values of the physical properties of the pump and the simulated vessels. The mechanical model has the important advantage of being homologous with its counterpart in a living system. Pressures are dramatically demonstrated by the heights of columns of fluids, pulsations can be seen to be a function of the stiffness of the connecting tubing, and venous congestion is obvious behind a failing pump.

However, mechanical models do have their limitations in teaching situations. Their very mechanical nature imposes design constraints, fabrication costs, and the necessity for adjustment and repair. Their simplicity, while a virtue, also limits their realism and accuracy. Once designed and built, the scope of a mechanical model is apt to be fixed without provisions for expansion and increased realism.

## MATHEMATICAL MODELS

The virtues and the hazards of using mathematical models is a continuing debate in physiology. Those individuals originally trained in the physical sciences accept mathematical models as a concise way to codify facts and as a mechanism for predicting performance under new circumstances. Others often prefer to think in terms of direct experimental observations without precise abstractions. This book does not attempt to enter the argument head on, but rather to illustrate that mathematical models provide reasonable facsimiles suited for teaching demonstrations. Perhaps familiarity with such successes will dimish the resistance to quantitative models for a few without extingishing the healthy skepticism which we all should retain.

It is very difficult for the human mind to keep track of several interacting variables as they change with time. When these interactions can be accurately formulated computer models provide greater insight than can be achieved by intuitive arguments. It would seem that holistic models, such as Dr. Dickinson's respiratory model and Dr. Guyton's cardiovascular model, will eventually be subjected to enough scrutiny that their limitations will be established. Once this stage is reached, if not already, there are tremendous teaching benefits to be derived from subjecting inanimate mathematical formulations to stresses and observing the homeostatic responses.

Once a research model has been formulated, tested, and accepted there is every reason for putting it to use in teaching situations which stay within the limitations of the model. This seems to be the case for the Hodgkin and Huxley model for excitation in the squid axon, a concept which has persisted in our textbooks for over 25 years. This involves empirical formulations for the time- and votage-dependent changes of membrane conductances. A computer simulation based upon the formulations for sodium and potassium currents following a stimulus provides students a wealth of insight about the properties of excitable tissue and the proposed mechanism for its threshold. There is no chance that the casual student can duplicate the experimental skills required in the original experiments. Just as he/she may read in depth about established facts it seems that students should also be presented the opportunity for the unique insights gained from working with simulations. In so doing this does not have to preclude their exposure to experimentation; it is just that this experimentation can not explore the accumulation of past accomplishments.

Most physiologists have an intuitive appreciation for algebraic expressions but many are refractory to equations which include rates of change. The very essence of physiology includes body compartments whose contents are in a continual state of flux. The variables may be in a steady state described by algebra but more often there are fluctations introduced by environmental changes, ingestion and fasting, and physical activity. The equations describing the variables under these circumstances include gains and losses which are changing with time and thus form differential equations. Formal courses in differential equations are not common in the training of physiologists. This is partly because of the theoretical approach of most such courses but also because practical problems in physiology contain nonlinearities which can not be solved analytically. Thus there is often some doubt about the relevance of the analytical approach. The accessiblity of personal computers and their ability to provide iterative solutions to such problems may have long-range effects upon the attitudes of future physiologists.

---

ANALOG COMPUTERS

---

One method of solving differential equations by computing equipment uses electrical voltages as analogs directly proportional to the variables in the equation. Electronic "operational" amplifiers are combined with resistors and capacitors so that their output voltages are proportional to the time integral of their input voltages. For example, in the solution to a simple first-order decay problem, in which the rate of decay is proportional to the amount which remains, a fraction of the output of the electronic integrator is used as the input. The choice of the size of the resistors and capacitors determines the simulated rate of decay.

Analog computers have generally been replaced by digital computers, for reasons to be discussed below, but there are many advantages to working with analog voltages. Any analog model consists of many operational amplifier integrators all acting instantaneously and in parallel. This gives a very real gain in computation speed when compared with digital solutions which perform integrations one at a time over finite time intervals. The speed combined with the ability to change parameters by changing the values of one or more variable resistances permits the operator to gain a "feel" for how the total system responds to disturbances.

Analog computers have been used extensively for physiological simulation, both with research and teaching objectives. The "chemostat" model for respiration of Grodins et al (1954) used analog computer techniques to model the ventilatory response to inhaled carbon dioxide. Chapter 7 of this book cites a reference to Dr. Bolie's analog model of the glucose-insulin interaction. There have been many others, particularly during the midcentury years before the availability of digital computers.

Beeuwkes and Braslow (1971) designed a preprogrammed analog computer model of the cardiovascular system which was later manaufactured by the Harvard Apparatus Company of Cambridge, MA. This Cardiovascular Analog Trainer (CAT) uses meters and dials calibrated in physiological terms such as circulating volume, venous tone, ventricular inotropy, and of course, pressures and flows. One of the features of this model is the ability to plot ventricular pressure-volume curves during changes in contractility and valvular lesions.

The reader is referred to the paper by Dr. Peter Stewart (1979) which makes a case for analog computation as a teaching adjunct in physiology. One of his points is that it is much easier to create a voltage analog than a mechanical one; it substitutes mental effort for machine shop materials and skills. In that recent paper he identifies the components of an analog computer and illustrates its use in a respiratory model which controls carbon dioxide.

In spite of certain intrinsic advantages of analog computation the trend is toward digital computation. This pace is apt to be accelerated as microcomputers become personal possessions just as analog machines once were. Analog computations achieve their greatest potential when some of the variables in the model are already voltage analogs, as the outputs from flow and pressure transducers. However if one is working entirely from mathematical equations digital programming in an algebraic-based language such as FORTRAN or BASIC seems more natural. The necessity to convert mathematical relationships into corresponding electrical interconnections is awkward for the person without experience in electronics. The variables must be scaled to provide voltages within the range of +/- 10 volts and the units of time have to be scaled to provide solutions within a reasonable time. This can be a formidable task in very large models. The setting of the parameters and the readout of the solutions are limited in precision to the order of 1 part in 1,000.

## DIGITAL COMPUTERS

During the last 20 years there has been increasing use of institutional macrocomputers and departmental minicomputers for digital simulation of physiological models. Most of these applications have been associated with research projects but in many cases the models also have been used in the classroom (DeLand, 1978). Professor James Spain (1979) of Michigan Technological University has prepared a teaching manual, Basic Computer Models in Biology, a preliminary version of an introductory textbook. Although the formulations involve differential equations and flowcharts rather than specific computer listings, the examples range from biochemical kinetics to ecological systems and are intended to introduce biology students to applied mathematics. Professor Spain stresses the pedagogic value of having the students develop their own models rather than using "canned" programs.

Computer-aided instruction (CAI) is a general term which includes mathematical simulation but, more frequently, the term implies a method of presenting students with questions followed by a set of alternative answers. The programmed logic branches according to the selected answer, either supplying further drill on the questioned concept or advancing to the next level. Many of these programs keep track of the progress of individual students and the frequency of the respective responses. The hardware requirements for this application include a keyboard and printer or CRT for each student and a large data storage facility. Generally this is achieved by many operators time-sharing a large central computer which may be used for a large number of different applications.

One of the most advanced time-sharing instructional computers is the Programmed Logic in Automatic Teaching (PLATO) developed at the University of Illinois in Urbana and now maintained by Control Data Corporation. There is a vast network of terminals at colleges and universities throughout the middle western states which use an extensive library of teaching programs written by experienced teachers. One main feature of the installation is the high-resolution of the CRT display and the ability to project slides onto the screen for even finer detail. A paper by McKown and Barr (1973) in The Physiologist illustrates the display for neuron electrophysiology, even to the point of simulated placement of the electrodes into the cell. The resulting membrane conductances, currents, and voltages are computed using the Hodgkin and Huxley model.

Starting in 1975 technological developments placed so-called microcomputers on the market at costs ranging from $500 to $5,000. Since this is the approximate initial investment for acquiring terminals which access time-shared computers it is expected that many of the functions formally handled by sharing one marcocomputer will gradually be shifted over to self-contained microcomputers. Although there will be a continuing need for large computers, there are many advantages to transferring more trivial operations to dedicated machines.

The present book stresses microcomputer applications in physiology where solutions to differential equations are presented as graphs on the CRT screen. In teaching applications the speed of displayed computations is important since the student may have to run through several settings of any one parameter in order to understand the role of that parameter. Such computations may be done precisely and rapidly in a macrocomputer but the results are typically communicated to the remote terminals at either 10 or 30 characters per second. This delay, unreasonable in certain situations, is completely eliminated if the simulation is done in a self-contained computer. The essence of interactive simulation exercises demands rapid response of the computer to actions initiated by the student. Since time-shared systems have response times which are a function of the number of users on the system at any one time, this can be a serious problem.

There are many intangible personal benefits to having convenient access and control of a piece of equipment, either for teaching or for research. Microcomputers are portable and can be carried to the lecture room, discussion group, and library without concern for telephone connections and the administrative logistics of a shared facility. It is anticipated that personal computers will become as commonplace as slide projectors but supply programmable displays which are much more flexible in format than those on films. The subject of this book is to illustrate the hardware required and the range of applications in teaching a first course in physiology.

```
TEACHING BY SIMULATION
```

The last two chapters of Dr. Dickinson's book discuss the use of interactive simulation models in teaching within physiological and clinical settings using the respiratory model outlined in the first of his book. The present book contains chapters devoted to several different models as used by the author in the teaching of physiology. In most cases these are devoted to simple but basic concepts which can be illuminated by on-the-spot graphic displays.

These models are used first as a demonstration during the lecture, using standard large-screen video monitors which are common in modern lecture halls. This is effective and adds excitement to the lecture almost without exception. The process of choosing and entering the parameters and then the following of the plotted solution, point by point, gives a sense of active participation far beyond that of drawing a curve on the chalkboard or projecting a static view from a slide. Such facilities may become common in future lecture halls.

Involvement in individual self-study exercises is not universally successful in that many students in biology have a natural resistance to anything tainted with mathematical overtones. The secret of overcoming this prejudice lies in the ability of the programmer to couch the simulation in realistic terms. Dr. Guyton tells the story about the medical student at his institution who became some so emotionally involved in an exercise that the student fainted when he was unsuccessful in overcoming a simulated irreversible phase of shock.

REFERENCES

Beeuwkes, R., and N. Braslow: The cardiovascular trainer: A real time physiological simulator. Physiology Teacher 3:4-7 (1971).

Deland, E. C. (Ed.): Information Technology in Health Science Education. New York: Plenum Press (1978).

Dickinson, C. J.: A Computer Model of Human Respiration. Baltimore: University Park Press (1977).

Grodins, F.S., Gray, J. S., Schroeder, K. R., Norins, A. L., and Jones, R. W.: Respiratory responses to CO-2 inhalation. A theoretical study of a non-linear biological regulator. J. Appl. Physiol. 7:283-308 (1954).

McKown, R., and L. Barr: Simulation of excitable membrane experiments. Physiologist 4:658-668 (1973).

Modell, M. I., Fahri, L. E., and Olszowka, J. J.: Physiology teaching computer simulations--problems and promises. Physiology Teacher 3:14-16 (1974).

Spain, J. D: Basic Computer Models in Biology, Houghton, MI: Mich. Tech. Univ. Book Store (1979)

Stewart, P. A.: The analog (computer) as a physiology adjunct. Physiology Teacher: Physiologist 22:43-47 (1979).

Tidball, C. S.: Affirmation of conventional physiology laboratory exercises. Physiology Teacher: Physiologist 22:25-26 (1979).

Chapter 2

MICROCOMPUTER COMPONENTS


The microcomputer market is characterized by its variety
of manufacturers, models, and options. Therefore it seems
necessary to give some preliminary introduction to the hardware,
software, and operating systems themselves before proceeding to
the simulations. Such background material has to be superficial
but the intent is to emphasize the features which are
significant in selecting and using a microcomputer for teaching
simulations. More detailed information is obtainable from
operating manuals and manufacturer's literature.

This chapter outlines the major components in a
microcomputer system. The next discusses programming languages
and operating systems highlighting the features of each which
are important to our present discussion. This is followed by a
chapter which describes two hardware enhancements essential for
effective simuation applications; namely, high-resolution
graphics and the use of a numerical processor for computation
speed. Chapter 5 describes three different microcomputers used
by the author for the simulations in the balance of the book.
These are considered to be representative of the different
models on the market today.

Figure 2.1 diagrams the important components of a
microcomputer system and serves as a focal point for the topics

James E. Randall, Microcomputers and Physiological Simulation

in this chapter. The microprocesser, or central processor unit (CPU), is the brain of the design and the "bus" serves as the peripheral nervous system communicating with the effector organs. The CPU provides signals on control lines to initiate data transfer to or from the listed devices selected according to the binary-coded combination of signals on the address bus lines.

As an example, the CPU may identify a keyboard by a specific coding of the address bus lines. At that time the value of a pressed key may be transferred on the data bus lines into the microprocessor where it later may be returned to some other address identified as memory, printer, or mass storage. Each of these categories will be described in a general way. At the end of the chapter there is a listing of the addresses of the manufacturers cited.

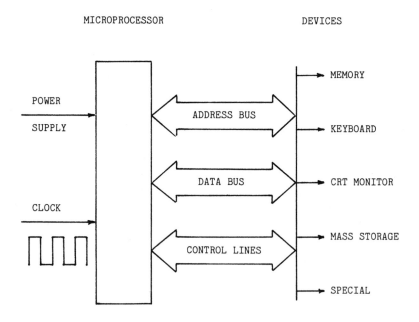

Figure 2.1.  Components of a microcomputer system.

## MICROPROCESSSORS

Most people are familiar with the impact that the replacement of vacuum tubes with transistors has had upon our society, providing small electronic devices which use less power as typified by transistor radios. Some fewer persons may be aware that "integrated circuits" combine the function of several discrete component transistors, resistors, and capacitors into a single "chip" with perhaps 14 or 16 pins. For a time these were the building modules for computers in that they performed logical operations such as providing a voltage at one pin depending upon whether there was a voltage or no voltage present at each of other pins in some particular combination.

The next stage in technical development came with large-scale-integration (LSI) technology where the functions of thousands of transistors are combined into a single package the size of a large postage stamp. Such a chip is at the heart of the pocket calculator supplying all of the functions except for the keys and the numerical display in a single package that can be mass-produced with minimal expense for labor.

Microprocessors are another example of the marvels of LSI. Instead of gaining flexibility by the manner of interconnecting a large number of fixed logic integrated circuits these new devices are few in number but depend upon software programming to adapt the internal logic to the needs at hand. Not only is the size of the unit reduced but mass production reduces the hardware costs replacing them with the labor of writing the programs (software) to execute the needed logic. Consumer appliances are beginning to replace mechanical timers with the more reliable and more flexible microprocessors so that engineers must now know not only about digital logic but also how to program these devices.

Two of the first microprocessors were the Motorola 6800 and the Intel 8080, either of which can be purchased now for less than $10. The Z-80* has enlarged the 8080's instruction set and is used in many of the microcomputers available today, e.g., in the Radio Shack** TRS-80**. The Intel 8085 contains hardware improvements but uses the same instructions as the 8080. Software written for the 8080 can also be run on the 8085 and the Z-80. The 6502, made by MOS Technology, is used in the Apple*** II and other microcomputers.

---

\*    Z-80 is a registered trademark of Zilog Inc.
\*\*   Radio Shack and TRS-80 are registered trademarks of Tandy
       Corp.
\*\*\* Apple is a registered trademark of Apple Computer Inc.

There are other microprocessors in use, each with their own advantages and advocates, and the number is continually growing. Arguments can be made for the relative merits of each but for the purposes of this book, where a whole computer system is under consideration, the way any microprocessor is integrated into an overall sytem should be the major consideration.

Microprocessors typically are 40-pin integrated circuits with pins used for power supply, a clocking signal, address lines, data lines, and control lines. Except for the power supply the voltages which appear at these pins follow binary transistor-transistor-logic (TTL) with a voltage near 0 being considered as a logical 0, or low state; a voltage near +5 volts is considered a logical 1, or high state. The purpose of the balance of this section is to describe some of the functions that occur at these pins.


CLOCK FREQUENCY

One method of classification considers the frequency of the timing signal called the clock. Most commonly this is either at 2 MHz or 4 MHz with respective periods of 500 and 250 nanoseconds as the minimum time for the computer to perform internal operations. For example, the simplest instruction, called a "no op" or NOP, requires several clock cyles to access the memory and then increment the program counter within the microprocessor. A more involved operation where data were being moved from one memory address to another requires correspondingly greater time to execute.

Operationally the higher speed is useful in repeated computations, as encountered in simulations, but at the same time the electronic circuitry may be more critical and fast-access memory is more expensive. These possible limitations are becoming less critical so that 4 MHz microprocessors are worth serious consideration.

It should be noted that the 6502 microprocessor has a "look ahead" feature so that every clock cycle can be a memory cycle. In effect this increases execution speed by anticipating the next memory location while still processing information taken from the present one.


WORD SIZE

The number of pins allocated for data and instruction transfers between the microprocessor and the rest of the computer is another method of classification. Most commonly 8 pins are allocated for this purpose with the 8 logic levels (bits) being referred to collectively as a "byte". This 8-bit word size provides 256 different combinations of binary configurations starting with 00000000, 00000001, ..., on through 11111111. Although the logic uses the base 2 it is more common to describe the numbers using shorter notations such as octal (base 8), hexadecimal (base 16), or decimal (base 10). BASIC typically uses the convenience of decimal notation but anyone who does any assembly language programming with microcomputers will have to become used to the inconveniences of hexademical notation where the 16 digits used are 0, 1, 2, 3, 4, 5, 6, 7, 8, 9, A, B, C, D, E, and F. As an example, the hexadecimal equivalent of decimal 255 is the two digit number "FF" corresponding to (15x16)+15.

The 8-bit word size, offering only 256 different combinations of 0's and 1's, imposes a constraint on applications limited to one word. The new generation of micropocessors coming on the market now have 16-bit word size and thus offer greater instruction flexibility, greater computational resolution, and improved memory management rivaling the large minicomputers. At the same time the greater flexibility and applicability means greater complexity so it seems that the 8-bit microcomputer will remain in use for some time to come. The alternative approach is to combine two or more 8-bit words so as to increase the number of possible instructions and the numerical resolution. This is done at the expense of computation speed because the microprocessor can transfer only one 8-bit byte at a time.


MEMORY ADDRESSING

Typically, current microprocessors have 16 pins allocated for selecting one of 65,536 different binary combinations starting with all pins low (0) and ending with all pins high (1). These select memory locations for which the data byte may be transferred to or from memory storage circuits or peripheral devices. It is convenient to refer to these 16 bits in terms of a LOW byte (the least significant) and a HIGH byte (the most significant).

For example, when the programmer wishes to load the microprocessor accumulator with a byte from a given 16-bit memory address he presents the microprocessor with an operation code (OP CODE) consisting of three bytes, each presented in succession through the 8 data pins. The first byte is a code for a LOAD ACCUMULATOR, the second gives the low byte of the address, and the third the high byte of the address. More advanced microprocessor internal architecture provides for speeding repeated operations but the programmer using a language such as BASIC is not aware of these internal details.

The manner by which groups of bytes are combined to give greater resolution to data is of concern to the programmer. One should be aware of integer and floating point numbers, or in the nomenclature of FORTRAN, integers and reals. Typically integer data, such as for the subscripts of variables in arrays, use two bytes in most 8-bit microprocessors.

Floating point, analogous to scientific notation, typically uses 4 or 5 bytes; one for the exponent of two, the remaining 3 or 4 for the mantissa in binary format. These can give precisions of either 6 or 9 decimal digits, respectively, sufficient for teaching simulations in most cases. It should be pointed out that some programming languages achieve greater precision than either of these only with significant costs in computation speed and storage space.


INPUT/OUTPUT PORTS

Communications of bytes of information between the microcomputer and external devices, such as keyboards, printers, CRT displays, or numerical processors, may be achieved by allocating one or more memory addresses for this purpose. Special logic decodes the one address and activates the device permitting transfer of a byte into or out of the microprocessor data pins. This method, called memory-mapping, is that used with the 6502 and 6800 microprocessors.

Alternatively, the 8080/8085 and Z-80 microprocessors leave all of the 65,536 addresses available for memory uses by incorporating specific instruction codes which provide an additional 256 addressable input (analogous to reading memory) and output (analogous to writing into memory) ports. At specific times during these I/O instructions 8 of the address pins contain the binary logic for one of the ports and additional pins indicate whether data is to be transferred into or out of the microprocessor on the data pins. One of the sources of incompatibility between different microcomputer configurations is that of having devices assigned to different I/O ports and thus requiring modification of software written for one configuration before it can be used with a different one.


SEMICONDUCTOR MEMORY

At one time computers stored binary numbers in minute magnetic rings with the direction of the magnetic flux lines distinguishing between a 0 and a 1. More recently large-scale-integration (LSI) provides the equivalent of thousands of transistors on a single integrated circuit chip arranged in combinations permitting the storage of large amounts of binary information in a small package at low cost and requiring simple circuitry for accessing this information. The manufacturing processes are improving continually so that each year it is possible to get more bits into each chip at a lower cost per bit (currently about one cent/byte). Since the amount of information in a memory chip is going to be some power of two it is common practice to refer to multiples of 1,024 rather than of 1,000. For example, the currently popular size stores 16K (16,384) bits. This section indicates some of the general features of semiconductors memories which are of concern to anyone using microcomputers.


ROM


        The one major disadvantage of semiconductor memory is that when the power is removed and reapplied the logical states come back in an unpredictable pattern bearing no relationship to the information placed in them initially. However, there are special designs, called ROMs for read-only-memory, which can be permanently programed to contain always the same information. These are useful in microcomputers to initialize an operating system when the power is first turned on or for dedicated applications.

        One popular microcomputer, the TRS-80, has BASIC in about 12K of ROM which is available immediately upon turning on the power switch. In the case of teaching simulations it is likely that once the programs for exercises have been refined they can be placed in ROM, perhaps upon a plug-in module, eliminating the cost and inconvenience of a mass storage device. This is the philosophy of the Texas Instrument model 99/4 microcomputer introduced in 1979.


RAM


        To distinguish it from the ROM version the more common memory is called random-access or RAM. Typically 8-bit microprocessors use memory chips in multiples of 8 with each chip in the group being assigned to one of the bits in the data word. Thus a chip storing 4,096 (=$2^{12}$) bits will have to have 12 address pins to pick the address of the data bit. These pins ultimately connect back to the least significant 12 address pins of the microprocessor and determine the location for information transfer on the data pins of the memory and microprocessor.

        Since the microprocessor has a total of 16 address pins the remaining 4 determine which of the 16 possible 4K groups is being addressed. This is achieved by a logical decoding circuit

which activates a "chip enable" pin on the memory  chip.   Other
pins,  besides those supplying power, include one for inputing a
data  bit  into  the  location  being  addressed,  another  for
outputing stored data from the address determined by the address
pins, and finally a pin whose logical state (0 or  1)  indicates
whether the data is being read or written.

## DYNAMIC RAM

       As  more  information  is  stored  in  small spaces heat
dissipation becomes an important consideration.   One  kind  of
memory design reduces the power requirements and heat generation
significantly  by,  in  effect,  applying  the  power  only
intermittently.   These  so-called  "dynamic  memories" require
special circuitry to refresh repeatedly the logical states which
otherwise  gradually decay with time.  Timing of this process is
critical and often  microcomputers assembled from components  of
several  different  manufacturers  may  not function as a system
though they are faultless in other configurations.   Because of
their  efficiency  and  low  cost,  currently about $100 for 16K
bytes,  dynamic  memories  are  used  in  most  single-unit
microcomputers, such as the TRS-80 and the Apple II.

## KEYBOARD

       The  keyboard is required for entering and debugging new
programs and  for  student  interaction  with  the mathematical
models.    It  may be combined with a printer, housed within the
microcomputer itself, or in a separate case.  Because it is  the
one  component  which receives hard physical use in the hands of
students the mechanical and electrical design  must  be  sturdy;
otherwise errors and erratic performance will gradually develop.

       The  keyboard  transfers  alphanumeric  and  control
characters  into  the  8 data pins  of the microprocessor when
accessed  by  decoding  circuitry using  the  I/O  port  (or,
alternatively,  memory  address) commands.  Since the characters
are  coded in binary logic there is the  potential  for  $2^8=256$
different  combinations.   Those which are printable include the
alphabet starting with the upper case letter A which is coded as
a  binary 01000001 according to the so-called "ASCII" code which
is given in most computing manuals.

       The  control  characters, obtained  by  pressing  an
auxiliary key and a letter key simultaneously, are used for such
functions  as  momentarily  halting the simulation in process or
starting another one.  The method of correcting bad entries,  as
by  a  delete key or backspace, varies among different keyboards

so this function, and the other control functions should be well
identified or explained for the new operator. Lack of skill of
simple operations, such as terminating a parameter entry with
the RETURN key (and not spelling out the letters R-E-T-U-R-N),
is part of the reason for the common barrier to the use of
computers. Good designs with obvious means of starting the
system and parameter entry are critical elements in having
computer simulations accepted as a teaching tool.

```
┌─────────────────────────────────────┐
│  CATHODE RAY TUBE DISPLAYS           │
└─────────────────────────────────────┘
```

        Along with the economy of microprocessors and
semiconductor memories, the use of commonplace TV rasters for
display of computer output contributes to the low cost of
microcomputers. Besides the advantages of cost, quiet
operation, and mechanical reliability the cathode ray tube (CRT)
display provides features not attainable by a printer. Most of
the latter operate at speeds of either 10 or 30
characters/second, a rate which can be tedious to follow in
reading as the information is transferred from the computer. On
the other hand operating instructions, questions, and options
can be transferred almost instantaneously to the CRT in a manner
analogous to turning the page of a book. This feature may not
seem important to the dedicated operator but it can become
crucial in seeing that the technique is used by a student who
may already be sleepy and bored by the subject at hand.

        The other feature which makes the CRT particularly
useful is its ability to present graphic displays as dynamic
variables change with time. Of course any program development
requires printed output so a possible arrangement is to have one
printer accessible to the instructor for programming and keeping
grade records, while other microcomputers use only the CRT
output for student applications.


TV RASTER

        The economy of the CRT display system used in
microcomputers arises from the standardization and mass
production of television sets. These, or preferably video
monitors, can be be used with microcomputers for either color or
black and white displays of computer output. The devices use a
standardized "raster" in which the CRT electron beam sweeps
across the screen line by line and from top to bottom. The
video signal intensifies the beam at each position on the screen
according to the image being transmitted. The nature of the TV
raster imposes certain limitations on computer displays, but the
alternatives cost an order of magnitude greater.

RESOLUTION

For convenience in discussion consider the  screen  as  a
matrix  of  small  dots,  called  "pixels";  the number of these
elements which can be displayed on  the  screen  determines  the
resolution of graphs, the detail of alphanumeric characters, the
characters/lines and the number of lines on  the  screen.    The
vertical  resolution  is  set by the 525 lines displayed on  the
screen every 1/30th second.  The microcomputer must generate and
supply  a  "composite"  video  signal containing synchronization
information that starts the vertical raster and each line in the
raster  and  also  modulates  the  intensity  of  the  dot as it
traverses the screen on a given  line.    Since  the  horizontal
sweep rate is at 15.75 KHz, with 57.8 microseconds available for
display on each sweep, the number of discernible dots across the
screen will be determined by the ability of the intensity signal
to turn off and on during  that  57.8  microseconds.    This  of
course  is  dictated by the bandwidth of the signal as generated
in the computer and transferred by video circuits to the CRT.


MONITORS

Best horizontal resolution is  achieved  using  a  video
monitor;  currently  it is possible to purchase a 9" model which
has 600 vertical line resolution with a bandwidth  of  about  10
MHz.    The small size gives crisp characters which can be viewed
at close distances consistent with the size of the computer  and
keyboard  placement.    A slightly more economical alternative is
the use of a television set but this arrangement  requires  some
mechanism  for  getting the computer-generated signal to the CRT
in spite of the fact that the normal input to a television is  a
radio  frequency  (RF)  signal  being  modulated  by  the
synchronization and video intensity  information.    One  method
involves  a modification which bypasses the RF input and channel
selection circuits, placing the computer signal directly at  the
CRT.    Since  many  economical  TV  sets  do  not  have  power
transformers there is a problem of isolating the circuit  ground
from the power line.

Another alternative is to provide  a  "modulator"  which
would allow the computer to modulate an RF carrier equivalent to
channels 3 or 33.  This arrangement is  convenient  to  use  and
requires  no TV modifications but the quality of reproduction is
compromised.  Also  such  modulators  are  in  effect  miniature
transmitters with the potential of interference to other sets, a
point  of  current  concern  to  the  Federal  Communication
Commission.    Instructors should be aware that many lecture room
monitors  require  an  RF  input.    It  is  projected  that  as
microcomputers become more commonplace a direct video input will
be a standard feature of all television sets and thus allow  one
CRT to serve both educational and entertainment functions.

MEMORY REQUIREMENTS

     Besides the constraints of the CRT monitor  itself  other
factors  must  be  considered in display designs.  These include
the amount of memory utilized for holding the information  being
displayed  on  the raster and the logic circuitry which converts
stored information over to a signal which intensities the CRT at
the correct times on the raster.  As the number of characters or
graphic resolution increases the  memory  dedicated  to  display
goes  up  as the product of horizontal and vertical resolutions.
If color is added this increases the storage requirement.

     Presently  there is considerable flexibility and variety
in the options for converting stored information into  character
and  graphic  displays.   As  the  demand  for  higher  graphic
resolution, intermixed graphics  and  alphanumerics,  and  color
displays  increases  there  will  be  improved  designs  at more
reasonable prices.  A common format of display  is  to  have  64
characters  on  each of 16 lines which requires a total of 1,024
8-bit bytes of memory to store them.  The option of 20 lines  of
80  characters  each is useful for text editing but puts greater
demands  upon  the  quality  of  the  video  montitor.    Many
inexpensive  computers  use  either 32- or 40-character lines to
economize upon the memory requirements and the CRT quality.

     Alphanumeric  information  is  stored in memory in 8-bit
bytes according to the ASCII code; for example the memory mapped
onto a blank display screen may be filled with the binary number
00100000 corresponding to the  code  for  a  space.  Entering  a
letter,  such  as A, is done by filling one memory location with
its ASCII code.  Typically the characters  are  displayed  as  a
matrix of 7x9 dots on a 8x16 cell (to allow for spacing) so that
for 16 lines of 64 characters the required resolutions would  be
256  vertical  by  512  horizontal,  achievable  with good video
designs.  Options available,   depending  upon  the  electronic
circuitry, include upper and lower cases and special symbols.

     Out of the 256 different binary codes possible with the
8-bit  number  up  to  128  are  assigned  to  characters.   The
remaining bit may determine whether  a  displayed  character  is
white  on  black  or  black  on  white,  or may even provide for
user-generated  symbols.   The  TRS-80  achieves  its  graphic
displays  by  having  the  most  significant  bit  turned  on to
indicate that the low 6-bits are not to be considered  as  ASCII
code  but  rather  as  identifying  the on or off status of 6 dots
arranged in a 2x3 matrix at a  screen  location determined by  the
memory location.

SERIAL VIDEO TERMINALS

     The  present  discussion  of  cathode  ray tube displays
applies to those which  are memory mapped,  having a design with

close coupling between the microprocessor, the memory, and the CRT interfacing circuitry. Another possible arrangement is to use a CRT terminal as a peripheral device addressed through one of the microcomputer I/O ports. In that version serial strings of binary-coded impulses are decoded into alphanumeric characters by the CRT electronic circuitry. In general there is greater utility and economy in incorporating the CRT interfacing into the main computer and then using a simplier video monitor or a modified TV set. This permits the use of memory for either program text or CRT display. The external CRT terminals are useful additions when one wishes to have a large number of upper and lower case letters on the screen, as in word processing of manuscripts, without impinging upon computer memory.

Because of the importance of graphic displays in the general plan of this book we shall return to this topic in a later chapter discussion of enhancements for simulation applications.

## MASS STORAGE

Since programs are lost from conventional semiconductor memory when the power is turned off it is imperative to have some alternative means of storing the large variety of routines which any one computer may use. The usual procedure in microcomputers is to have a simple operating system stored in ROM which starts automatically when the power is turned on. This can then be used to "bootstrap" more complicated routines in from a storage medium. There are two general kinds of mass storage used with microcomputers: conventional audio tape cassettes are inexpensive but slow and of marginal reliability to use; flexible magnetic disks (called "floppy" disks) are much faster and more reliable, but also more expensive.

### AUDIO CASSETTES

The more economical microcomputers store operating systems, high-level interpreters, and user programs on the familiar Phillips-type audio cassettes using inexpensive recorder/reproducers. The computer must contain circuitry to code binary numbers into a string of audio-frequency tones or pulses that will be recorded on the magnetic medium. Upon playback the computer must do the reverse process, but be tolerant of the fluctuations in tape speed, noise, and differences in amplitude that are characteristic of this mass-produced equipment. The tape speed of 7.5"/sec fixes the maximum rate of magnetic flux reversals and thus the maximum rate of transfer of binary information between the tape and the computer. Much effort has gone into developing schemes which will approach the theoretically limiting rate but 1,200 bits/sec seems to be the practical limit.

For computers which already have BASIC permanently on ROM the user´s particular program can often be read into memory within less than a minute; but the loading of programs requiring thousands of bytes of memory (the computer may have up to 64K bytes) can take a very tedious amount of time. For the first year of his class use of microcomputers the author was limited to cassettes for mass storage and the simulation of the Hodgkin and Huxley equations, which was then in 20K of memory, took 4 minutes to load from tape. He found this to be tolerable as long as that was the only program to be loaded during a lecture or to be used by students on a particular day. It would be intolerable for running many different programs at one sitting -- no student would finish the set.

Besides putting the binary information onto tape the computer must have software routines to know where to get or put the bytes in memory, how many to transfer, and some rudimentary way of checking whether the numbers read from the tape match those which were put on to it originally. There are many different ways of formatting this information so that audio tapes from one kind of computer may or may not run on another type.

Because of the large number of certain kinds of microcomputers, such as the Radio Shack TRS-80, the Commodore PET*, and the Apple II, commerical software and software exchange is common within each of these types. Outside of this group there is a format initiated by some of the first microcomputer hobbyists at a meeting in Kansas City which sometimes is used for exchange purposes but its 300 bits/sec rate is too slow for routine use. There are others, but unfortunately no one is really usuable by more than a minority of the microcomputers on the market today.

Audio cassette storage is apt to remain popular with the person who is purchasing a microcomputer with personal funds but their inefficiency makes them a poor investment for the institution which is serious about teaching by simulation. During the program development stage disks, described below, are much more practical. Once exercise software has been fully developed it can be more economically and conveniently stored on plug-in ROM modules when large numbers of student stations may be involved.

---

* PET is a registered trademark of Commodore Business Machines

FLOPPY DISKS

        The serious use of microcomputers in business
accounting, word processing, and scientific applications
requires rapid access to large programs and data files which can
conveniently be called into memory by name as given in a
directory. The development of flexible magnetic disks costing a
few dollars each and using hardware costing from $500 to $2,000
places these small computers into competition with the large
time-shared configurations. Anyone who has graduated from audio
tape to disk storage will never be willing to revert back -- it
is a quantum jump in efficiency in programming and operation and
should be argued vigorously as an investment in productivity.

        The one disadvantage of disk storage is that there have
been several physical ways of putting the information onto the
magnetic material and of formatting the starting addresses,
number of bytes, and checking transfers so that there are now
some 5 or 6 popular forms of disk storage. This is another
inhibiting influence upon the exchange of software. There are
four components to be considered in regard to discussing these
alternative designs: the magnetic disk itself, the drive unit
which rotates it, the controller which converts binary
information over to signals to locate and energize the recording
head at the disk, and the software which orders the binary
numbers into some format.

        Floppy disks (diskettes) rotate within a square
protective jacket and have the general appearance of a 45 rpm
record in its wrapper. They come in two sizes, those which are
in 8-inch square jackets were first. Then came the
"mini-floppy", in a 5.25-inch jacket. The former, being first,
have the advantages of precedent, large capacity and rapid
access time. Both versions record the information in
concentric circles called "tracks", further broken into arcs or
"sectors". The larger disks are usually formatted according to
the IBM 3740 standard which has 77 tracks with 26 sectors for
each track for a total capacity of about 250K bytes. This
"single density version" is one of the more common methods of
interchanging disks between different microcomputers,
particularly for those using the so-called CP/M operating system
which will be described in a later chapter. It is now also
possible to obtain a "double-density" large floppy with a
capacity of about 500K bytes.

        The compact and economical mini-floppies appear to have
adequate capacity for teaching needs. However, there are
several formatting methods which preclude free interchange of
all disks of this size. One classification scheme is based upon
the method of locating the beginning of a given sector on a
given concentric track. In the "hard sector" versions there are
physical holes at the beginning of each sector, these provide a

positive identification as they rotate past a hole in the jacket and allow a light beam to be sensed by the electronic circuits. In the "soft sector" versions there is only one hole to indicate the start of a track, the location of individual sectors must be done by software which senses identifying markers within the track.   An additional difference involves the density of recording on the disks which means that there will be different storage capacities.

The original mini-floppy design was by Shugart Associates with single density and soft-sector formatting.  This was used in a popular disk system known as North Star, one of the more common formats for microcomputer programs from suppliers.  More recently North Star has doubled this capacity from 90K bytes to 180K bytes. Micropolis, perhaps second in popularity of the mini-floppies, has two versions of hard-sector diskettes.   That with quad-density has 77 tracks of 16 sectors with 256 bytes/sec for a total of about 315K bytes; another version has 35 tracks with 135K bytes on the same size disk. Just now these are popular but with the recent addition of disk systems for the inexpensive TRS-80 and Apple-II lines their respective formats may become widely used also.

The details of drive units, electronics, and controllers do not need to concern us here.   A later chapter will be concerned with disk operating systems, another point of diversity. Since this section has a decidely pessimistic taste regarding the compatibility of different disk systems it might be wise to interject a note of perspective. We are just now at the beginning of a process of hardware evolution that has made tremendous progress in the relatively short time of less than four years.   As far as hardware for teaching simulations are concerned (and probably all other applications as well) we are still in a period of experimentation and growth.  It will be some time before a particular configuration emerges as "everyman's simulator".  In the meantime there are opportunities for us all in influencing the direction for the future.


WINCHESTER DRIVES

Large computer installations use 14-inch rigid magnetic disks for rapid access to large amounts of data.  In 1979 a number of manufacturers introduced an 8-inch rigid "minidisk" based upon the same Winchester drive technique. Units selling for less than $2,000 can store about 11 megabytes.   For reliability and speed the units have nonremovable disks so that they are intended for information of an archival nature.

This is an important development for increasing the utility of small computers but it is not particularly important for mathematical simulations for teaching purposes where

convenience of transporting programs is more important than mass
storage. The floppy disk is still the appropriate media for
teaching exercises.

---

```
┌─────────────────────┐
│  MICROCOMPUTERS     │
└─────────────────────┘
```

     The start of the popularity of personal microcomputers
is credited to an article in the January 1975 issue of Popular
Elecronics which featured the Altair*. This was a kit costing
less than $400 which included the microprocessor, front panel
with toggle switches and lights for examining memory and
entering programs, cabinet, and 256 bytes of memory. The
manufacturing firm, MITS of Albuquerque, had anticipated about
500 orders but soon found them numbering in the thousands so
that prolonged backorders were not uncommon. MITS has since
become incorporated into a larger company which no longer sells
that computer, but one feature left its mark, the Altair bus,
now called the S-100 bus.

     The bottom of the Altair consists of a "mother board"
with provisions for up to 16 100-pin sockets connected in
parallel as a "bus". This serves as a method of mounting and
interconnecting a wide variety of computer modules according to
standardized pin connections. For example, one plug-in board
interfaces the microprocessor; another holds the memory;
another can interface I/O devices such as CRTs, printers, and
tape cassettes. Specific lines are assigned specific functions,
such as 16 of the 100 connect the address lines from the
microprocessor central processor unit (CPU) to the memory;
others supply the clock signals that synchronize functions with
the CPU cycles; and two sets of 8 handle the data into and out
of the CPU data pins.

     This was originally a "standard bus" simply because it
had no competition at the time; it did not arise from trial and
error so its faults have been subjected to much criticism. But
the fact remains that a small industry grew up supplying
special purpose interfacing cards for the S-100 bus. Now one
can purchase single boards holding 64K bytes of memory, disk
controller interfaces, assemblers on ROM, voice synthesizers,
and assorted graphics generators.

     Other computers also use the S-100 bus, but in slightly
different ways so that not all plug-ins are compatible in all
combinations. Some computers which are not based upon this bus
can be supplied with adapters to make use of the full range of

---

* Altair was a registered trademark of MITS, Inc.

the hardware available. Many of the small firms supplying these
special products have gone out of business but the S-100 bus
still provides the greatest range of hardware options and
software of any of the personal microcomputers on the market
today.

Later manufacturers felt that the cost of S-100
connectors, which could total to as much as $100 in a complete
configuration, and other features were not warranted and
consequently there became a number of alternatives each striking
out in new directions. One of the first ones was the Commodore
PET which has BASIC on ROM and a built-in CRT and tape cassette.
Many other computers have their own internal bus structures
making it possible to add on special units from a variety of
sources.

Because of the large number of possible combinations of
microprocessors and peripheral devices computer hobbyists are
producing a wealth of magazine articles on this subject. In
1979 two major firms, Texas Instruments and Hewlett-Packard, are
slated to enter the consumer computer market so the alternatives
are still increasing. At the same time a number of the early
microcomputer manufacturers are no longer in business. As was
the case with pocket calculators, marketing and business
management skills may be more important than engineering design
for the survival of individual microcomputer models.

After a discussion of programming languages and
desirable hardware additions, Chapter 5 describes the three
computer configurations used in the simulations given in this
book. As a way of illustrating the components described in this
chapter it can be noted here that all three use 8-bit data words
and 16-bit addresses. The keyboard and interfaces for CRT
monitor and audio cassettes are an integral part of the
microcomputer on each. Disk drives are possible additional
options.

The TRS-80 uses a Z-80 microprocessor with 2 MHz clock,
dynamic memory chips, and memory-mapped input/output ports. The
CRT has 16 lines of 64 characters each and requires hardware
modification for lower case characters. The Apple II uses a
6502 with 1 MHz clock, dynamic memory, and memory-mapped I/O.
The CRT displays 24 lines of 40 characters and lower case
characters are obtained with special software. The SOL-20* uses
the S-100 bus and has an 8080 microprocessor with 2 MHz clock
frequency. The display has 16 lines of 64 characters with upper
and lower case being a standard feature.

---------------

* SOL-20 is a registered trademark of Processor Technology, Inc.

REFERENCES

        In an endeavor that just began 4 years ago and which  is
changing  very  rapidly there are few landmark references.  When
computers  cost   hundreds   of   thousands   of   dollars   the
manufacturers  were  able  to  supply  extensive  consulting and
literature but when the total  cost  is  $1,000  the  purchasers
often have to seek the detailed specifications on their own.

        The best sources of information on  microprocessors  and
microcomputers  are presently in the articles and advertisements
in several computing hobby magazines,  such  as  Byte,  Creative
Computing, Interface Age, Kilobaud Microcomputing,  and Personal
Computing.  The publishers of these are listed  at  the  end  of
this  chapter.  There are also newsletters, many specializing on
specific  computer  models.  Microcomputer  literature  may   be
difficult  to locate in libraries but recent copies of magazines
can be found in retail computer  stores  which  also  provide  a
selection of manuals on both hardware and programming languages.
The managers of these stores can be very helpful about selecting
hardware   but   they  may  not  appreciate  fully  the  special
requirements  of  scientific  applications.      Most   academic
institutions  seem  to  have  people familar with microcomputers
located in the physical science departments.

        The  following articles and paperback books are possible
sources in addition to the manufacturer´s literature.

An Introduction to Microcomputers, Volume 0: The Beginners Book,
Berkeley:  Osborne & Associates Inc. (1976)

An  Introduction  to  Microcomputers,  Volume 1: Basic Concepts,
Berkeley:  Osborne & Associates Inc. (1976).

Barna,  A., and D. I. Porat:  Introduction to Microcomputers and
Microprocessors, New York: Wiley-Interscience (1978).

North,  S.:    Personal  computer  comparison  chart.   Creative
Computing 5:30-31 (Nov. 1979).

Poe,  E.  C.,  and  J. C. Goodwin, II: The S-100 and other Micro
Buses.  Indianapolis: Howard W. Sams, Inc. (1979).

Shipton,  H.  W:  The  microprocessor,  a  new  tool  for   the
biosciences.  Ann. Rev. Biophys. Bioeng. 8:269-286 (1979).

Waite,  M.,  and M. Pardee:  Microcomputer Primer.  Indianapolis:
Howard W. Sams, Inc. (1976).

## MICROCOMPUTER PERIODICALS

Byte Publications Inc.
70 Main St.
Peterborough, NH 03458

Creative Computing
P. O. Box 789-M
Morristown, NJ 07960

Interface Age
Published by McPheters, Wolfe & Jones
16704 Marquardt Ave.
Cerritos, CA 90701

Kilobaud Microcomputing
Published by 1001001, Inc.
Pine St.
Peterborough, NH 03458

Personal Computing
Published by Benwill Publishing Corp.
1050 Commonwealth Ave.
Boston, MA 02215

## MANUFACTURERS CITED

Apple Computer, Inc.
10260 Bandley Drive
Cupertino, CA 95014

Commodore Business Machines
901 California Ave.
Palo Alto, CA 94304

Hewlett-Packard
11000 Wolfe Road
Cupertino, CA 95014

Intel, Corp.
3065 Bowers Ave.
Santa Clara, CA 95051

Micropolis Corp.
7959 Deering Ave.
Canoga Park, CA 91304

MANUFACTURERS CITED (Continued)

MITS, Inc.
Albuquerque, NM 87106
In 1977 purchased by Pertec Computer Corp.
21111 Erwin St.
Woodland Hills, CA 91367

MOS Technology, Inc.
Valley Forge Corporate Center
950 Rittenhouse Road
Morristown, PA 19401

Mostek, Inc.
1215 W. Crosby Road
Carrollton, TX 75006

Motorola Semiconductor Products, Inc.
P. O. Box 20912
Phoenix, AZ 85036

North Star Computer
2547 Oakmead Parkway
Sunnyvale, CA 94086

Processor Technology, Corp.
7100 Johnson Industrial Drive
Pleasanton, CA 94566
(Not in business in September 1979.)

Radio Shack Division of Tandy Mfg., Inc.
1300 One Tandy Center
Fort Worth, TX 76102

Shugart Associates
435 Oakward Parkway
Sunnyvale, CA 94086

Texas Instruments, Inc.
P. O. Box 1443
Houston, TX 77001

Zilog, Inc.
170 State Street
Los Altos, CA 94022

Chapter 3

OPERATING SYSTEMS AND PROGRAMMING LANGUAGES


No collection of computing hardware can function without a list of logical instructions, a program. There is an abundance of microcomputer hardware but a shortage of software tailored specifically for each of the wide variety of potential applications. Indeed, the intent of this book is to stimulate such an activity for the purpose of teaching physiology.

Operating systems are programs used for such things as saving a part of memory on a diskette and placing its name in a directory so that it can be loaded simply by name for use. Programming languages are conveniences for deriving the logical instructions used by the microprocessor from statements or commands having some relationship to mathematical formulae or English words.

The first microcomputers used front panel switches to examine and modify the contents of memory and to start programs. Later versions contained "monitors", permanently stored in ROM, with which an operator could examine memory by entering the address on the keyboard and viewing its contents on the CRT display. In the more recent models turning on the power switch automatically starts a ROM-based BASIC, even loading and executing a program through the disk operating system (DOS).

The purpose of this chapter is to highlight the particular programming methods used in later chapters. The

James E. Randall, Microcomputers and Physiological Simulation

discussion is based upon 8-bit microprocessors having 16-bit
addressing capabilities, such as the 6800, 8080/8085, Z-80, and
6502, the most popular versions in use at this time. The SOL is
used as an example of the general class of S-100 microcomputers.
The popular TRS-80 and Apple II offer additional illustrations.

## MONITORS AND OPERATING SYSTEMS

    The distinction between a monitor and an operating
system is fuzzy but the main function of the monitor program
often is to provide access to the computer memory and its
Input/Output (I/O) accessories. The original Altair contained a
collection of toggle switches and a set of lights connected to
the 16 address lines and 8 data lines of the S-100 bus as a
method of examining and modifying memory contents at locations
addressed by the binary combination of switch settings. In some
cases "bootstrap" programs consisting of many steps had to be
toggled in by hand in order to provide the computer with the
capability of loading programs from mass storage devices.

    This mode was popular with only the technical hobbyist
so modern microcomputers perform these functions by using the
keyboard and the CRT through monitor routines either permanently
on ROM or callable from a disk. To reduce their memory
requirements these use coded letters as commands and hexadecimal
(base 16) numbers for addresses and data bytes. This requires
some computer jargon for the person who initializes the computer
configuration but not for the student operator.

    As an illustration, the SOL computer has a
monitor/operating system, called SOLOS, which is started
automatically when the power is turned on. This is in the
computer on ROM starting at the beginning of the last 16K of the
possible total of 64K of memory. It may also be restarted at
any time by hitting a particular combination of two keys on the
SOL keyboard. When started this monitor responds with a ">" as
a promptor on the CRT screen. Commands allow dumping the memory
onto the screen or printer, entering values into memory,
changing the output from CRT to printer, and saving or loading
parts of memory on tape cassette.

    The student wishing to load a program into the SOL from
a disk enters a command such as ">EX F400". This then executes
a routine on ROM starting at hexadecimal location F400 (decimal
62,464) which brings in a disk operating system (DOS) from disk
and starts it. From that point on all communication is in
English words or phrases and decimal numbers so that the need
for jargon is very small.

In the case of the TRS-80, turning on the power starts the computer in BASIC using it as a monitor or operating system. The commands PEEK and POKE can be used to examine or change specific locations in memory; other commands transfer programs between memory and disks; still others permit branching to non-BASIC routines in upper memory. This and several other computers seek to put the operator in immediate communication with the high-level programming language without the special knowledge which can be a barrier to computer use. In principle any computer can be designed to be self-starting for a dedicated task, such as a teaching simulation. The advantage of monitors is that they provide greater flexibility for different combinations of hardware units.

The Apple II can be configured to turn on in either the monitor mode or in BASIC. When power is turned on to models equipped with the Autostart ROM the disk operating system is initialized and the first BASIC program on the disk is executed. This can give operating instructions and call other programs, such as individual simulation exercises. (See the illustration on page 227.) In the other option the computer is initially in the ROM-based monitor. This provides features for the technical user, including a rudimentary assembler (see a later section of this chapter), a simple disassembler, and provisions for single stepping through a machine language program. Communication is provided between BASIC and the monitor, but the automatic starting feature is clearly desirable for student-operated microcomputers.

Generally "operating systems" are much more sophisticated than monitors and include special software required for accepting ASCII characters from the keyboard, sending such characters to the CRT or printer, and transferring programs and files between memory and the mass storage medium. SOLOS on the SOL and BASIC on the TRS-80 and Apple II performs these functions with audio tape in economical installations.

Disk operating systems (DOS) maintain directories listing files and programs callable by name. In the previous chapter the diversity of formats for floppy diskettes was emphasized. This mass storage comes in two different physical sizes; several methods of identifying where bytes start on a sector within one of the concentric tracks; and single or multiple densities of recording. This means that each particular kind of disk has to have its own software for locating the recording head over a track, for counting the number of bytes in a sector, and for allocating disk and directory space.

In practice each disk manufacturer supplies its own operating sytem so that the user can immediately load utility programs and high-level programming languages, such as BASIC. A functioning DOS and selection of programs gives a competitive edge in a market offering considerable alternatives. Some of these place their systems in the lower part of memory and run the programs in the upper part; others do the reverse. Each DOS has its own special way of formatting the disk files, assigning directory space, and utilizing common subroutines. This means that programs written to run under one DOS may not be used on another DOS even if the microprocessors have the same operation codes and the diskettes the same physical formatting -- yet another source of incompatibility.

---

> ## CP/M

As with many microcomputers, the Apple-II and TRS-80 have their own disk operating systems which are not compatible with any others. Each of these machines is popular enough that there is a large amount of software available on their respective disk systems. Another popular form of disk-based programs uses the operating system called CP/M*, an attempt to achieve software compatibility for machines having different hardware configurations. This system permits the programmer to ignore the details of the particular microcomputer being used and instead communicate with the system CP/M which has been tailored for that hardware. CP/M is a common method of distributing word processors, BASIC, FORTRAN, and other software on disks for the S-100 bus microcomputers.

This system functions with any microcomputer using the 8080/8085 or Z-80 microprocessors and having at least 16K of memory. It is available on a variety of floppy disks formats, including the IBM, North Star, Micropolis, Helios, and (with modifications) the TRS-80. In fact, one firm, Lifeboat Associates of New York City, makes a business of supplying versions which will run on each of the more popular disk drives and also supplying utility programs which operate within the framework of this operating system. Thus CP/M is becoming the common denominator between a variety of 8080-type microcomputers and disk units.

Being modeled after the DEC-10 System found in computer centers it offers powerful flexibility in combining and transferring files between disks and the CRT or printer. However, setting up a given memory and I/O configuration for CP/M for the first time requires technical knowledge and diligent attention to a set of obscurely-written manuals. Once this initial hurdle is over, or bypassed with assistance, it is

---

* CP/M is a registered trademark of Digital Research.

a very logical and convenient system to operate. Again, the
difficulties are encountered by the programmer, not by the
student who only has to type in a single title like SPIKE to
load and start the program on simulation of the action
potential.

The original version of CP/M was designed around the
8-inch IBM format floppy disk by Professor Gary Kildall doing
business as Digital Research in Monterey, CA. The currently
available manuals are written for this disk. Versions for other
disks, those supplied by Lifeboat Associates, have "disk
drivers" programmed specifically for the respective disk units
and which, in many cases, take 2K or 4K more of memory for the
DOS. These also require supplementary information about how to
initially set up the mini-floppies. Once these are in place
programs will run the same on any microcomputer running with
CP/M as long as they are contained within certain memory
boundaries.

All versions of CP/M use the first 256 bytes of memory
(first "page") when starting up or when a program must refer to
the operating system for disk operation. The first locations
contain information identifying where the rest of the operating
system is located and which devices are assigned for input and
output uses. The last 4K to 8K of memory is assigned for the
operating system itself so that a given configuration is valid
for up to a certain limit of memory but no more. The
recommended minimum memory for serious CP/M use with BASIC is
32K; with FORTRAN it should be 48K. In CP/M, programs are moved
onto disk starting from decimal memory location 256; similarly
programs which are loaded from disk must also start at that
location. If a program in memory no longer needs access to CP/M
the first 256 locations are available so that there are schemes
for running programs designed on other systems to start at
location 0.

CP/M has five console commands in memory for listing the
disk directory, erasing files from it, renaming file names,
saving memory (starting at location 256) onto disk, and typing a
given file on the output device. The output device for these is
normally the CRT but the simple process of pressing the CONTROL
and P keys simultaneously turns on the printer when one is
available.

Other more extensive commands are called by name from the
disk either for programming applications or for simulation
exercises. Some of these are used to modify the system for
different amounts of memory, to edit and assemble machine
language programs, and to ascertain the space remaining on the
disk. One particularly powerful command is called PIP, for
Peripheral Interchange Processor. This permits transfer of one
or more source files to a designation such as a disk file,

printer, CRT, or even to a larger computer accessed by a MODEM.
PIP is particularly useful for combining a number of small
documents into one package.

     In summary, CP/M is suited for microcomputers using the
8080 instruction set (such as those with a S-100 bus) and a wide
range of software is available on the popular disk formats. The
initial adaptation of this system for a given set of hardware
components is fairly technical and requires knowledge of
machine-language programming. Also CP/M and the high-level
languages are all proprietary and must be purchased by anyone
who wishes to receive teaching exercises available in this
format. This software cost is significant even before the
simulations are obtained.


┌─────────────────┐
│   ASSEMBLERS    │
└─────────────────┘


     Writing programs in high-level languages, such as BASIC
and FORTRAN, is the most efficient use of programming time.
However, there are situations in which it is necessary to deal
with the lists of 8-bit instruction codes as they are actually
applied to the microprocessor in "machine language". This is
the case when a software program must be written to incorporate
a special printer into an operating system. Also there are
situations where computation speed is paramount so that it is
necessary to invest programming effort in order to avoid the
time consumed in having BASIC interpret English into machine
code during each interation of the simulation.

     For example, the graphic solutions of the Hodgkin and
Huxley equations for the action potenital require about 2-3
minutes to simulate 10 milliseconds of an action potential when
the program is written in BASIC. A numerical processor chip
(for speed in evaluating the many exponential expressions) and
machine language programming accomplishes this task in 10
seconds. The BASIC interpreter and program takes about 22K of
memory while the all-machine-language version can run in just
under 6K of memory.

     The original Altair had 16 toggle switches with which
the operator could set a memory address and then enter the 8-bit
machine codes in successive memory locations. This was tedious
work even for the 256 bytes of memory which came with the
machine. "Assemblers" are software routines which convert
alphanumeric mnemonics into microprocessor code. For example,
NOP, meaning no operation, is converted to 0 for the 8080; a JMP
ABC, meaning jump to location labeled ABC, will be decoded to
three bytes, one for the JMP and the other two to identify the
16-bit address of ABC. An "editor" is the software routine

which     accepts the programmer's list of mnemonics and comments
and then outputs the file used by the assembler.    Editors   are
also  useful for writing some forms of BASIC or FORTRAN, and for
the word processors used for manuscript editing.

        CP/M  comes  with  an editor and an assembler, but there
are more useful versions available.    The   existence  of  these
routines does not mean that they have to be used in order to use
a microcomputer or to do simulation.  In fact   for   the   popular
computers,  such as the Apple II, the PET, and the TRS-80, BASIC
is the main software and an assembler is considered an accessory
to be purchased by the computer specialist.


┌─────────────┐
│   BASIC     │
└─────────────┘


        The   usual high-level language for microcomputers is some
version of BASIC which contains an "interpreter"  which  accepts
statement  lines in succession and converts them over to machine
code as the program is run. Smaller in   number   are   "compiler"
versions  which  convert  the entire program to machine code and
save the latter in a compact form which can be run   much   faster
than  the  interpreter  versions.    FORTRAN is a more elaborate
compiled high-level language offering the   advantages   of   speed
and compactness.  On the other hand the convenience of debugging
the interpreter languages is a major  consideration  for  casual
programmers.

        BASIC was developed at  Dartmouth  College   in   1963  by
Professors  Kemeny  and Kurtz with the idea of placing computing
power into the hands of beginners.  There probably are at   least
25   dialects  of  this  language  sharing  an  "ANSI   standard"
vocabulary of certain words but  with  considerable  differences
among others.  The reader is referred  to  the  excellent  BASIC
Handbook written by David A. Lien, and  published  by  Compusoft
Publishing of  San  Diego,  California.  This lists each of the
BASIC words, gives examples of their use,   and   gives  practical
alternative  methods  of  achieving the same results in versions
which do not include the command or function.  The book does not
cover  the  control of peripheral devices, such as disks, tapes,
and printers.

        Some  versions  of  BASIC  are  particularly adapted for
business applications where, for example, there may be need   for
precision  running to 10 decimal places.  Certain of these store
the numbers internally in a  binary-coded-decimal  (BCD)  format
which uses  4  bits  of a data byte to code each of the decimal
digits: 0000 being zero, 1001  being  nine.    The  mathematical
functions,  such  as  addition and multiplication, operate upon
these  4-bit  entities  in  a way  that  can  provide   unlimited

precision at the expense of computation speed.  Most  of  these
are prohibitively slow for simulation applications.

        The original Altair BASIC was written  by  Microsoft,  a
firm  which  has  gone on to supply the most popular versions of
this language used in microcomputers today.  Microsoft BASIC  is
supplied in ROM with the PET, Apple II, and TRS-80 computers.  It
is available on both large and small floppy  disks  for  systems
using  CP/M.  These all permit the use of two-letter subscripted
variables whereas some  large-machine  verions  are  limited  to
single letters and digits.

        Besides its popularity there are additional  reasons  for
using  Microsoft BASIC in the simulation exercises in this book.
It stores its floating point variables in either 4 or 5 bytes in
a  format  which  is  very  similar  to that used by the Am-9511
numerical processor chip to be described in  the  next  chapter.
This  allows the programmer to use the conveniences of BASIC for
setting up parameters, such as stimulus amplitude and  duration,
where  speed  is  not  important.   Then these parameters can be
moved  to  machine  language subroutines using  the  numerical
processor  for speed.  As an example, efficient machine language
subroutines could be developed  which  would  do  time-consuming
tasks  which were of general applicability.  Teachers could then
design exercises in BASIC which would  determine  the  arguments
for the subroutines.  Such a scheme could give local flexibility
in  designing  teaching  protocols  without  the  necessity  of
bothering  with  the  details  of  the  more  technical kinds of
programming.

        The  four-byte format, called single precision, provides
up to 7 digits for the mantissa and an exponent between -38  and
+38.   The  floating point BASIC used with the Apple II (called
Applesoft) uses a five-byte  format  which  provides  9  decimal
digit  precision.   Either of these appears to be sufficient for
the teaching simulations.  All of these formats use binary,  not
BCD,  notation.   One  byte contains the exponent as a power of
two; the other bytes  contain  the  mantissa  normalized  for  a
minimum  decimal  value  of  0.5.   The  minimum  hardware
configuration supplied with  this  computer  contains  a  small
version of BASIC on ROM which handles only integer numbers.  The
floating point version, mentioned above, comes on tape  cassette
(from which it can be transferred to disk) or on an optional ROM
card.  Both the integer and the  floating  point  versions  have
free access to the DOS.

```
┌─────────────────────────────────────────┐
│   OTHER PROGRAMMING LANGUAGES            │
└─────────────────────────────────────────┘
```

The illustrative simulations used throughout this book are written in BASIC. This is because all present microcomputers use that as the primary high-level language and because its simplicity fits the introductory objectives of this book. Now that the market for microcomputer hardware has begun to stabilize somewhat there is increasing availability of other languages which offer advantages to experienced programmers.

PILOT is a language created at the San Francisco Medical Center specifically for computer-aided-instruction (CAI). It is much easier to program for question and answer material than is BASIC but it is not optimized for the computational requirements of those instructional simulations which are speed-limited.

FORTRAN is now available for systems using CP/M and for the TRS-80. This compiled language has the advantages of fast computation speeds and using less memory when compared to BASIC. Also, special machine-language subroutines, such as those for superimposing characters onto graphics, can be called from a library. Since there are several physiological simulations already written in FORTRAN, experienced programmers may wish to follow this route. For example, the book by Dickinson cited in Chapter 1 is a detailed documentation of a model for human respiration which is written in FORTRAN.

As hardware costs decline attention is turning to the fact that programming effort, debugging in particular, is becoming the expensive component in making use of a computer. Pascal, named for the mathematician, is a programming language written in the 1970´s which is considered by many to be a significant advance over FORTRAN which originated in the 1950´s. Pascal is a structured language which emphasizes program planning and organization. This disciplined approach reduces program debugging and updating time and realizes the full potential of the computer in a wide variety of applications. Although most microcomputers have Pascal capabilities the newness of this language and its demands upon the programmer make its use premature for most readers of this book.

FORTH is a programming language which offers computation speed and compactness approaching machine language coding but which is much easier to implement than by using assemblers. FORTH uses a "threaded-code" compiler which produces a run-time program consisting of a string of addresses. Each of these addresses refer to the routines which execute the operations defined in the source program. The operands for these individual routines are pushed onto a stack and the operations executed in a manner analogous to the reverse Polish notation used in the Hewlett Packard pocket calculators. Languages similar to FORTH are available which realize the advantages of a floating point numerical processor chip to provide rapid simulations of speed-limited exercises such as those for the cardiac action potential.

## REFERENCES

Barden, W.:  How to Program Microcomputers. Indianapolis: Howard W. Sams, Inc. (1977).

Dwyer, T. A., and Critchfield, M.:  BASIC and the Personal Computer, Reading, MA:  Addison-Wesley Publish. Co., (1978).

Foster, C. C.: Programming a Microcomputer: 6502, Reading, MA: Addison-Wesley Publish. Co., Inc., (1978).

Jensen, K., and N. Wirth:  Pascal User Manual and Report, New York: Springer-Verlag (1975).

Lien, D. A.:  The BASIC Handbook, San Diego:  Compusoft Publishing, (1978).

Miller, A. R.: CP/M: An 8080 Disk Operating System, Interface Age, Pages 156-162 (July 1978).

Moore, C. H., and E. D. Rather: FORTH, A new way to program a minicomputer, Astron. Astrophy. Suppl. 15:497-511 (1974).

## SOFTWARE SOURCES

Digital Research
P. O. Box 579
Pacific Grove, CA 93950

Lifeboat Associates
2248 Broadway
New York, NY 10024

Microsoft
10800 N.E. Eighth, Suite 819
Bellevue, WA 98004

Chapter 4

## HARDWARE ENHANCEMENTS FOR SIMULATION

The microcomputers on the market up to 1979 have been promoted primarily for business applications and for games. In the area of education the main use has been at the primary and secondary levels, mostly to acquaint young people with the logical structure of computer programming. Scientific applications, simulation in particular, may require faster computation speeds than are possible with the usual interpreter versions of BASIC. In addition, high-resolution graphic presentations of dynamic processes have greater educational value than do columns of numbers. This chapter discusses two hardware enhancements which improve the usefulness of microcomputers for physiological simulation.

One of the more exciting opportunities offered by microcomputers is that they can be used for generating graphic displays mimicing what might be measured experimentally with a chart recorder or an oscilloscope. To achieve good resolution and to compute the solutions in a reasonable time requires that the microcomputer have special hardware capabilities not found in all models. The most flexible approach is to use an S-100 bus computer and purchase special interfacing cards for the graphics and numerical processing hardware. However, this may be costly and inconvenient when contrasted to those models which have graphics with reasonable resolution integrated into a single system. This chapter discusses these alternatives in terms of the more popular options available in 1979.

James E. Randall, Microcomputers and Physiological Simulation

GRAPHICS

Any microcomputer can produce a rudimentary graph of
some kind just as a typewriter can plot functions with poor
resolution. The author initially used a CRT display having 16
lines of 64 characters to plot the amplitude of a computed
action potential as a function of time, using the "*" as points
on the curve. For this the vertical resolution was 5 mv and the
time resolution was 0.2 msec for a total span of 12 msec.

Subsequent models have supplemented text capabilities
with graphics under the control of BASIC without the need of any
special hardware. There are two general approaches, either
character generators or bit-mapping. Character generators are
commonly used to place ASCII-coded alphanumeric characters on
the CRT screen. The generator intensitifies the video beam at
just the right instants according to an 8-bit code representing
the displayed character. Since the ASCII code does not use all
of the 256 possible combinations of the 8-bit code many
generators fill in graphic symbols, such as lines and arcs. In
some microcomputers the operator can define his own symbols,
saving them in RAM. This scheme is satisfactory for bar graphs
and certain kinds of tracings but in general it is slow and
inconvenient to use for plotting mathematical functions.

In bit-mapped displays each bit in a section of memory
corresponds to a specific spot on the CRT screen. If the bit is
set (high or on) that dot is intensified; if it is off, the dot
is blank. For a screen with 256x256 resolution this requires
64K bits of memory, or 8K bytes, a significant amount.
Furthermore, if each dot is to have several levels of intensity
or different colors, the number of bits required increases
accordingly. Drawing a line on the screen requires a software
routine which locates the memory bits corresponding to the x and
y-coordinates for each point in the line. Text characters are
entered as dots in a 4x6, 5x7, or other matrix by software which
accepts a text string as an argument. The characters may be
defined in any configuration within the matrix by the
programmer.

It is not practical to expect microcomputers to
realize the full range in resolution, intensity, and color as
used in television viewing. For example, for 512 lines in a
frame with 512 dots each with 256 levels of color and intensity
requires about one quarter million bytes of memory for storing
this information. Professional computer displays use other
methods. The Tektronix 4051, which has a resolution of 1024
vertical by 784 horizontal dots, saves the image in the CRT
phosphor. The balance of this section describes the more
economical compromises of bit-mapped graphics as implemented in

three representative microcomputers which use conventional TV-type rasters.

## TRS-80

The CRT display for the TRS-80 microcomputer contains 16 lines of 64 positions at which either a text character or a 2x3 graphic matrix can be displayed. Each of these positions on the screen corresponds to a single byte of 1K of RAM memory. When the most significant bit of a given byte is off (equal to zero) that byte is used to convey an ASCII code. For example, if the screen is blank and in the text mode, all 1K bytes of the CRT memory buffer contain a decimal 32, the ASCII code for a space. If the most signficant bit of any memory byte is set (equal to one) the low 6-bits of that byte tell the display pattern of the 2x3 graphic matrix at the screen position mapped by the memory location.

This arrangement provides a vertical scale of 48 dots and a horizontal one of 128 dots. The individual dots are addressable by a BASIC command which can be placed within FOR ... NEXT loops to draw lines or functions. Each of the 1K positions on the screen can contain either a text character or a 2x3 graphic matrix so that labels can be intermixed with axes and computed solutions. Figure 12.2 (page 171) contains an illustration of an action potential computed and displayed on a TRS-80. The vertical resolution is 10/3 mv and the time span is 5 msec with 0.05 msec resolution.

## APPLE II

One of the attractive features of the Apple II is that it has a high-resolution graphics capability integrated into the BASIC by vector commands. This resolution is 192 vertical by 280 horizontal in black and white. Many of the illustrations in this book are photographs of this display. They have sufficient resolution to plot not only an action potential, but the stimulus and ion conductances as well. Colors are introduced at reduced horizontal resolution.

Out of the total of 64K of memory in the Apple two 8K segments are assigned to two different "pages" of high-resolution graphics, selectable by software. In addition, there is a separate portion of memory assigned for alphanumeric text. The software can switch between these three modes allowing display of the text, as for instructions or tabular data, and either of two different graphics panels. It should be noted that the 16K of memory used as a graphics buffer is also available for programs and data storage. There are circumstances in which both pages of graphics can not be used.

The command HCOLOR=Z sets the color for subsequent plotting commands according to the argument Z. HCOLOR=7 will plot white dots, HCOLOR=0 will erase them. Single dots are plotted by HPLOT X,Y in which X has the range 0 to 279 and Y has the range 0 to 191. The origin is in the upper left corner of the screen. Vectors are plotted by the command HPLOT X1,Y1 TO X2,Y2 ... TO XN,YN. Vertical and horizontal lines are a single dot wide or high but lines at certain angles appear fuzzy because the algorithm which connects the ends of these vectors fills in more than one dot at each abcissa position.

An entire 8K graphics buffer area can be stored on disk and recalled as a unit without having to generate the total field each time it is used. One demonstration disk distributed by the manufacturer, called a slide show, contains a number of digitized pictures which are clearly recognizable.

The intermixing of text and graphics in this microcomputer requires special mention. One of the pages of high-resolution graphics can optionally have 4 lines of 40 characters at the bottom of the screen. These lines can be scrolled and addressed by the usual PRINT statements to place running comments or instructions during the plotting of a function. In some of the figures of this book the author placed small letters on graphs by an expedient, but inefficient, method using the HPLOT vectors. A more eloquent method consists of temporarily replacing the usual PRINT implementation with a special binary subroutine which places printed text into the graphics buffer rather than into the text buffer. This routine and a character table, which may be defined with arbitrary letters and symbols, is loaded from disk at the start of the BASIC program. The required software is supplied by the manufacturer.

S-100 BUS MICROCOMPUTERS

Generally speaking, the use of graphics with S-100 bus microcomputers requires a custom-tailored hardware and software configuration. The hardware consists of a video interface board which plugs into the bus and drives a separate video monitor. Individual positions on the CRT screen may be addressed through I/O ports of the 8080/8085 or Z-80 microprocessor used with the S-100 machines. The BASICs used with these microcomputers can then do the plotting using the OUT A,B command where A is the port number and B is the x or y-coordinate to be intensified. This is an inefficient method for most plotting and text so that special machine-language rouines are required for drawing vectors and placing labels. Implementation of this into a BASIC or a FORTRAN system is an individual effort up to this time.

One of the first S-100 bus graphics interface boards was the ALT-256*256 made by Matrox Electronics Sytems (see address at the end of the chapter). This was used by the author for about a year and will be described as illustrative of this approach, though there are others on the market today. The Matrox board is bit-mapped and contains 8K bytes of dynamic memory which operates independent of the memory addressed by the microprocessor and thus does not slow down the computations as some alternative graphics boards have done. The resolution, with video monitors used in the United States, is 240 vertical by 256 horizonal.

The microprocessor communicates with this board by four successive I/O ports. When one output port is called the screen is blanked within 33 msec. Two others convey the x and y-coordinates according to the values 0-255 on the data bus. The display operation itself takes 3.4 msec to implement so that it is necessary to sample an input port until a previous display command has been completed. Once ready, an output on the fourth port turns a dot off or on at the coordinates previously transmitted.

The Matrox board supplies a composite output signal consisting of synchronization and video intensity information which goes to a video monitor. Unless special electronic design is involved this video output will be in addition to that supplied with the S-100 bus microcomputer for text. The author found it most economical and convenient to use two separate video monitors. The one connected for monitor and BASIC applications supplies the students with instructions and tabular information. The one connected to the graphics board supplies computed responses. The two 9" monitors sit side-by-side on the computer and provide simultaneous information of two kinds.

Subsequent to the Matrox 256x256 board there have been other graphics interface boards introduced upon the market. That manufacturer now has a 512x256 board which can give twice the horizontal resolution or rapid selection between either of two 256x256 displays. In addition it is possible to get 4 levels of intensity at each of 256x256 points. This board contains 16K bytes of dynamic RAM memory.

Newer graphics interface boards are approaching the resolution limits obtainable with commonplace TV monitors. It can be recalled from the discussion in Chapter 2 that the vertical resolution is limited by the 525 lines of the TV raster and the horizontal resolution is determined by the response of the electrical circuitry during each sweep of a line. The horizontal sweep rate is 15.75 KHz, defining the interval during which the intensity signal must turn off and on to display individual dots on the line. Typical monitors have a horizontal

resolution of 600 lines in the center of the screen and a
bandwidth of 10-12 MHz.

One of these S-100 interfaces, developed by Technical
Education Research Centers of Cambridge, Mass., is sold through
Cambridge Development Laboratory (address at the end of this
chapter). The display matrix for this board is 640 wide and 512
high and uses 40K bytes of on-board memory for the
single-intensity black and white configuration. For this fine a
degree of resolution the addressing of the x- and y-coordinates
requires multiple bytes on an 8-bit machine and thus can be
slow. The interface includes special single-byte control
commands to execute vector manuevers. For text displays the
interface has 80 characters in a 8x16 dot matrix on each
horizontal line. Special commands execute vertical scrolling of
text.

## NUMERICAL PROCESSORS

In many teaching simulations the effectiveness of the
exercise is severely compromised by the slowness of BASIC. This
is particularly the case in the computed membrane potentials
exercises which involve a number of time-consuming exponentials.
Programs written in BASIC may discourage students from making a
number of runs, as in establishing the chronaxie from a
strength-duration curve. There are many approaches to speeding
this process. Different microcomputers may have different clock
frequencies. The many versions of BASIC differ in their speeds.
Using compiler versions of BASIC, FORTRAN, or Pascal cuts out
the delays of interpreting each line of the source program as it
is executed. The chapters on action potentials indicate
numerical methods which provide improved accuracy with larger
integration intervals, speeding up program execution in this
way. The balance of this chapter describes a hardware
enhancement which can provide a speed improvement of ten times
when used with appropriate software.

"Numerical processor" chips are in effect preprogrammed
microprocessors which can perform mathematical operations and
evaluate functions once they have been issued the appropriate
command by the microprocessor. They in effect operate in
parallel with the main central processor unit and interact with
it only to be initiated and to provide the final answer. In the
meantime the main program can continue doing other things such
as plotting.

Most of these numerical processor chips have the same
computing potential as do the scientific pocket calculators.
Some of them are effectively revised calculator chips which are

inherently slow and which do not interface conveniently with 8-bit microprocessors. However, one of them, the Am-9511 Arithmetic Processing Unit, manufactureed by Advanced Micro Devices, Inc., does offer considerable computational advantages. The author has used this in the three representative microcomputers to reduce the time to simulate a 10 millisecond action potential exercise from 2 minutes in BASIC to 10 seconds using this chip with appropriate software.

## AM-9511 ARITHMETIC PROCESSOR UNIT

The Am-9511 Arithmetic Processor Unit, hereafter abbreviated as APU, is a 24-pin chip. Eight of these pins are connected to the microprocessor through the data bus. It is through this channel that 8-bit bytes of data, commands, or status information are transmitted between the APU and the central processing unit (CPU) microprocessor. The other pins supply power and clocking signals to the chip and also determine the intention of the information on the 8 data pins. Eight-bit input commands to the APU from the computer CPU determine the nature of the mathematical operation or function to be evaluated. Status information from the APU to the CPU tells whether the processor is busy or indicates error information, such as a division by zero.

Data transfer between the APU and CPU is in either two or four 8-bit bytes, depending upon the data format being used. Both 16-bit and 32-bit integer arithmetic is possible with this numerical processor but we shall limit our discussion to the 32-bit floating point operations. In this format one data byte represents the exponent of two, and the other three bytes give a 24-bit mantissa. In a manner very analogous to the reverse Polish notation on the Hewlett Packard pocket calculators the APU contains a set of internal registers called a "stack". This stack can hold four of the 32-bit (4-byte) floating point operands at any time. In use the CPU "pushes" each operand onto the stack in 4 single-byte operations. Then a coded command is issued to the APU by what is on the 8 data pins and the control pins. When the operation is completed, as indicated by status information sampled by the CPU, the answer is recovered by "popping" the corresponding four bytes from the APU stack and displaying or plotting it.

The speed arises from the fact that the CPU microprocessor has only to push the arguments onto the APU stack, issue one command for the mathematical function, and then pop the answers back out. This is a marked reduction in computation time when it is contrasted with the all-software versions which go through a multiplicity of operations, moving 8-bit data bytes in and out of the CPU. For evaluating an exponential the net savings in time are as much as 100 to 1.

There are, however, two prices which have to be paid. The 32-bit floating point format limits precision to between 6 and 7 decimal places, and the range is about $10^{20}$. In addition, input and output overhead reduces the realized speed advantage to more like 10:1 and requires appropriate software.

Microcomputers which use the Am-9511 require a special interface board which supplies the clock and power voltages and matches the commands and data transfers to assigned input/output ports. That is, an OUT N,X command can push the argument X onto the APU stack while an OUT N+1,Y tells the APU to treat the argument Y as a command. Input commands read either data from the APU stack or the current status. These illustrations could be executed with BASIC commands but to realize the full computing speed the communication between the APU and the CPU should be in machine language. The hardware and software requirements are now discussed for each of the representative microcomputers.


TRS-80

There is no commercially available product for interfacing the Am-9511 chip to the TRS-80 microcomputer. The main unit of this computer is the keyboard which contains BASIC on a ROM, 16K of RAM, and connections for power, audio cassette recorder, video monitor, and expansion hardware. The manufacturer's accessories which connect to the expansion connector include additional memory, printer, and floppy disk mask storage. As a demonstration project the author designed and built electronic circuitry which connects an APU chip to the TRS-80 bus through the expansion connector (Randall, 1979).

The demonstration software consists of a simulation of the Hodgkin and Huxley equations for a forcing by two separate stimuli with selected amplitudes and durations. Using only the BASIC this takes 90 seconds to simulate 10 msec. When the APU chip is used for the time-consuming parts this same simulation occurs in 15 seconds, faster by a factor of six. In this application BASIC is used to give the student instructions and to ask for stimulus parameters. Because of the similarity of the floating point format used by TRS-80 Level II BASIC and by the Am-9511 only a minor modification is required in order to have machine language subroutines do the actual "number crunching". This consists of evaluating the rate constants for the existing membrane potential, updating the dimensionless variables, calculating membrane currents, and then the new voltage. The voltage also is plotted while in the machine-language mode. Upon completing the final point on the plotted response, control returns to BASIC and asks for the next set of stimulus parameters.

This implementation requires both electronic and software skills but it does demonstrate what can be achieved at a modest cost for hardware.


## APPLE II

As of October 1979 there are two commercial interface boards available for the Am-9511 and the Apple II bus. One is manufactured by California Computer Systems (Model 7811B) and the other by Computer Station, Inc. (Fast Floating Point Board, or FFP). Their addresses are given at the end of the chapter. Each of these boards comes with a modified version of Applesoft II, the floating point BASIC used with the Apple II. In both versions the normal 9 decimal digit precision of Applesoft is reduced to between 6 and 7 digits and the range also is reduced. The precision is adequate for teaching simulations but there are situations where excessively small values of the rate constants of the cardiac action potential may give an error message. This can be avoided by prechecking those stages known to be vulnerable in the computation and providing alternatives.

The Model 7811B uses the Am-9511 for all floating point calculations whereas the FFP does all except the four functions since the overhead on these stages offsets any speed gained in the computation itself. Benchmark comparisons of repeated evaluations of an exponential show the speeds of these two boards to be similar in that application. The execution time is about 1/3 that for the same benchmark run with standard Applesoft. An action potential that requires 150 sec in standard Applesoft runs in 80 sec when the software floating point routines are replaced with the APU board.

This gain of a factor of two to three in computation speed is achieved using the same BASIC programming techniques with no need to resort to machine-language programming. It should be noted that the BASIC is loaded into the RAM area used as a buffer for one of the two pages of high-resolution graphics. This may require some minor modifications of programs which are written to run with the ROM-based version of Applesoft BASIC which resides in the upper 16K of memory.

In order to realize the full factor of ten potential gain in speed of the Am-9511 it is necessary to work with a programming language other than the interpretive BASIC. This can be done with assembly-language subroutines which get their arguments from the main BASIC program. Computer Station, Inc., which supplies the FFP board, has a "threaded-code" language similar to FORTH but which is designed to take full advantage of their APU interface board. FORTH is not used as commonly as BASIC but its reverse Polish notation approach is quicker to

implement than assembly language. In a benchmark program given
by the developer the Computer Station threaded-code language was
30 times faster than Applesoft without the APU.


S-100 BUS MICROCOMPUTERS

        In 1979 there is one commercial board for interfacing the
Am-9511 numerical processor to S-100 bus microcomputers.
MemTech Co. supplies this board with either a 2 MHz or a 3 MHz
processor chip. They can supply FORTRAN subroutines using their
interface board which will run specified benchmark programs 3
times faster. They have plans to release other software to
allow users to take advantage of the chip, including a version
of Microsoft's compiled BASIC. It should be noted that this
software is proprietary and must be purchased, both the original
high-level languages and the APU additions.

        The author has used the MemTech interface board with
machine language 8080 code to simulate 10 msec of nerve axon
potential in 10 seconds and to simulate the cardiac action
potential in 30 seconds. This is done by machine lanuage
routines called from BASIC with stimulus parameters as
arguments. Chapter 12 gives an example of how a BASIC program
is "human compiled" into a set of subroutine calls which
implement the numerical processor operations.

        Though the full implementation is too detailed for
presentation here the general approach of the machine language
subroutines is appropriate. A portion of memory is assigned as
a buffer for the floating point constants and variables used in
the simulation. The assembler assigns symbols, such as VOLTS,
to the addresses. Subroutines move floating point numbers from
these addresses into the APU stack, perform single numerical
operations as called in sequence, and then pop the result from
the APU stack back into a buffer address.

        The 8080 microprocessor internal register pair HL is set
to the address of the argument and a routine called PUSHFLT
pushes the argument onto the APU stack. Subroutines such as
EXP, MUL, and DIV are called to perform numerical operations
upon the arguments on the stack. These issue the appropriate
single-byte commands to the numerical processor chip, which
leaves the answer on its internal stack. Then, with HL set to
the memory address, a subroutine POPFLT pops the answer from the
APU stack into the buffer area of memory. Once the BASIC
program for the simulation is developed it is possible to mimic
it by a sequence of subroutine calls. This is a tedious process
to implement, but once done it provides rapid solutions of the
axon and ventricular action potentials.

REFERENCES

Randall, J. E.: Interfacing a numerical processor chip to the
TRS-80. Interface Age, 4:87-89 (1979).

Smith, D. G.: Apple II high-resolution graphics. Kilobaud
Microcomputing 33:104-106 (Sept. 1979).

Waite, M.: Computer Graphics Primer, Indianapolis: Howard W.
Sams and Co., Inc. (1979).

MANAUFACTURERS CITED

Advanced Micro Devices, Inc.
901 Thompson Place
Sunnyvale, CA 94086

California Computer Systems
309 Laurelwood Road
Santa Clara, CA 95050

Cambridge Development Laboratory
44 Brattle Street
Cambridge, MA 02138

Computer Station
#12 Crossroads Plaza
Granite City, IL 62040

Matrox Electronic Systems, Ltd.
2795 Bates Road
Montreal, Que. H3S 1B5, Canada

MemTech Co.
4891 Clairemont Mesa Blvd.
San Diego, CA. 92117

Tektronix, Inc.
P. O. Box 500
Beaverton, OR 97077

Chapter 5

REPRESENTATIVE MICROCOMPUTERS


This chapter is meant as a bridge between the previous three which provide technical background and the balance of the book which uses total microcomputer systems. The intent is to highlight the features of three representative microcomputers as an aid to anyone trying to decide upon the personal commitment and hardware required to set up a teaching simulation facility. The TRS-80 was chosen because of its initial low cost, national popularity, and widespread availability. The Apple II has good graphic resolution utilized by simple vector plotting commands in BASIC. Its convenient operating features and popularity makes it an attractive choice for teaching exercises which are to be exchanged between different institutions.

Greatest flexibility in selecting hardware enhancements and software systems is offered by microcomputers which use the S-100 bus. Lack of compatibility between different configurations may exclude software exchange. In 1977 the author chose the SOL-20 but its manufacturer went out of business in 1979. Its features still are representative of other models still in production and the estimated 200,000 S-100 units that are said to have been produced since the introduction of the Altair in 1975.

The author acknowledges that subjective opinion and chance played strong roles in selecting these particular models in a dynamic market but he thinks that all three are representative of the those on the market in 1979.

James E. Randall, Microcomputers and Physiological Simulation

TRS-80

The minimal configuration consists of a keyboard,  video
monitor,  and  audio  cassette  recorder/reproducer.  This can be
purchased for less than $1,000 in 1979.  The  keyboard  cabinet
contains  the  Z-80 microprocessor, 16K of memory, BASIC on ROM,
and interfacing circuitry  for  the  CRT  display  and  for  the
storage  of  data  and  programs on the tape cassettes.  There is
also a 40-pin connector for expansion interfacing to  additional
hardware.   Turning  on the power switch starts the computer in
Level II  Microsoft  BASIC  permitting  the  operator  to  write
programs or read in previously written ones from tape.

The Z-80 is capable of addressing  a  total  of  64K  of
memory.   The first 12K are dedicated to the ROM-based Level II
BASIC.  The next 4K are used for assorted functions  such  as  a
memory-mapped  keyboard  and CRT display buffer.  The 16K of RAM
is  available  for  BASIC  programs  and  variables  or  machine
language  routines  accessed  by BASIC.  This memory is adequate
for most of tabular simulations given in this book.

The  biggest  limitation of this modest investment is the
graphic  resolution  which  is  48  vertical  positions  by  128
horizontal  ones.   The  points  on the screen are individually
addressable by the BASIC command SET X,Y where the origin is  in
the  upper  left  corner.  Lines  can  be  drawn by placing this
command within FOR ... NEXT loops.   Text  and  graphs  can  be
intermixed conveniently.  Only upper case letters are used.

The addition of numerical processors or  high-resolution
graphics requires custom designs through the interface connector
on the rear.   There are conversion units which permit addressing
S-100 bus cards through this mechanism but they are not standard
and require electronic skills to implement and use.

The  intent  of  the expansion interface connector is to
connect Radio Shack accessories, such as a floppy disk, printer,
or  additional  memory.  The TRS-80 floppy disk operating system
is popular enough that there are several software sources  which
supply  word  processors, FORTRAN, and Pascal for this computer.
The CP/M option is available but since  its  standard  operation
conflicts  with  the  ROM  containing  BASIC  either software or
hardware  modifications  are  required  to  run   the   software
developed  for  other  kinds  of  hardware.   For  example, all
programs always start at location 256 for CP/M.   To  run  on  a
standard  TRS-80  these  would  have  to be relocated to RAM.  A
hardware modification is possible which  permits  the  Z-80  to
address either RAM or the BASIC ROM at the lower addresses.

The second model of the TRS-80, introduced in 1979, expands the mass storage capacity for business software but does not add graphic or "number crunching" capabilities as required for scientific computations and simulations. The 16K version with Level II BASIC is suited for personal purchases in which tabular results or low-resolution graphics are satisfactory.

## APPLE II

The standard configuration of the Apple II is illustrated in Figure 5.1. This consists of a keyboard and console, disk drive unit, and a video monitor. Rear connections are provided for the monitor and for recording and playing back on audio tape cassettes. The motherboard contains a 6502 microprocessor and a standard 16K of memory. There are provisions for bringing the total RAM up to 48K at a modest increment in price, an investment which is strongly recommended. The final 16K of memory contain ROM with a monitor and either of two versions of BASIC. The efficiency of the switching power supply reduces the cabinet weight to 11 pounds and eliminates the need for a cooling fan.

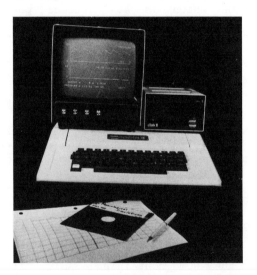

Fig. 5.1. The Apple II microcomputer, disk drive, and video monitor. Besides the keyboard the computer contains the microprocessor, 48K of RAM memory, and 8 sockets for interfacing modules. The pictured flexible diskette is 5.25" in diameter and stores over 100K characters, about two times the size of all of the programs listed in this book.

The   ROM-based   software   monitor   program   is meant for
technical users and includes a limited assembler,  disassembler,
and   memory   move and dump commands.  The keyboard is limited to
upper case letters and the screen has 16 lines of 64 characters.
Word   processor   applications   can   be done by using an external
video terminal with 24 lines of 80 characters.

Eight   50-pin   connectors   along   the   rear   of   the
motherboard   provide   opportunity   for   interfacing   peripheral
devices   to   the   bus.      For   example, one disk controller card
occupying one of the 8 slots can control two disk drives.      One
disk   drive   is   sufficient   at   a   student   station but two are
convenient for copying one disk to  another  in  order  to keep
backup   copies   of   software.    Other interfacing cards commonly
used are to drive a printer, a video terminal, MODEM to a larger
computer, or a numerical processor board.

In the minimum configuration  one  of  two  versions  of
BASIC   exist   in   the   ROM   in   upper   memory.   "Integer BASIC"
provides some graphics  capabilities  and  access  to  the  disk
operating   system   but   lacks   the   numerical   computation power
required for simulations.   The   other   version,  Applesoft   II,
provides   9-digit   precision   floating   point   arithmetic   and
high-resolution graphics commands.   Considerable   software   is
available for both versions of BASIC so it is wise to have both.

One approach is to have Integer  BASIC  on  ROM  on  the
motherboard   and to call Applesoft from disk.   This is necessary
when using the   numerical   processor   boards   with   overlays   as
described   in   Chapter 4.    This method has the disadvantage that
the disk-based Applesoft occupies the second 8K of RAM and  thus
prevents   the   use   of   one   of the two pages of high-resolution
graphics.

An   optional   firmware   (ROM)   card containing Applesoft
BASIC can be plugged into the first bus interfacing slot.      This
provides   instant   access   to either version of BASIC by enabling
either of two sets of ROM, one at time.   This leaves all of  the
bottom   48K   of   RAM   available   for   display buffers  and user
programs, but it also precludes certain uses  of  the  numerical
processor.      In order to do these it is necessary to remove the
firmware card from the first slot and depend upon  a  disk-based
version   of Applesoft specially written to take advantage of the
floating point   functions   on   the   Am-9511.      Having   hardware
floating   point   arithmetic   integrated   into   BASIC is a major
advantage for gaining speed during repetitive  computations,  as
during axon and ventricular action potentials.

An   Autostart ROM provides   several   conveniences.      For
student   applications   this   feature   comes into action when the
power switch is turned on.  This loads the disk operating system
and   automatically   starts   the   first   program   on the disk.  See

Figure 14.1 which shows a possible display, a "menu" of exercises which the student selects by number. Another feature permits a student to press the RESET button at any time in order to restart either the current simulation or return to the menu. Program editing conveniences also are included on the Autostart ROM.

A major advantage of Applesoft BASIC is that it permits addressing single points of the screen or drawing lines as vectors. The graphics features are described in the previous chapter but these include placing a dot at X,Y by the command HPLOT X,Y. The command HPLOT 0,0 to 100,100 draws a line using these pairs of numbers as coordinates on the screen. A disadvantage of this BASIC is that there are no formatting options for PRINT statements. The programmer has to use the integer function and powers of ten to print the desired precision of a variable.

Because the Apple II is widely used there is extensive software tailored specifically for its hardware and disk operating system. Since it does not use the 8080 microprocessor code there is no CP/M, nor is there a FORTRAN available. Instead, Apple has introduced Pascal as the sophisticated language for using relocatable machine language subroutines. Word processor applications require additional hardware to provide lower case characters and more than 40 characters per line on the CRT screen.

The disk operating system loads and runs binary routines, integer, and floating point BASIC. The names of the files and programs may be as long as 32 characters, a convenience for giving descriptive titles to exercises. A special EXECute command permits a disk file to perform operations as though they were being entered by an operator from the keyboard, a convenience for batch-processing certain kinds of programs.

In summary, the major feature of the Apple II is that it permits interactive graphic simulations in an integrated system which is conducive for widespread circulation of teaching exercises. In addition there are hardware floating point processors which provide speed advantages for programs written in BASIC.

## S-100 BUS MICROCOMPUTER

In spite of the short life-time of many of the
pioneering manufactures of S-100 microcomputers those models on
the market now are worth consideration by anyone who wishes to
do simulation using a personal computer in a serious way. These
provide considerable computing power at modest price. They tend
to appeal more to the person with previous experience on
marcocomputers than to those who have a rather causual interest
in microcomputing.

An S-100 bus requires a motherboard with several 100-pin
connectors and a power supply. Functional components, such as
the microprocessor and ROM-based monitor, may be either on the
motherboard or occupy one of the bus slots. Other units include
the memory, video monitor and disk controllers, keyboard and
printer interfaces, and special enhancements such as graphics
and numerical processors. Because the S-100 bus is meant for
8080/8085/Z-80 microprocessors CP/M is a common operating
system. This provides a wide range of software packages,
including FORTRAN, Pascal, and compiled BASIC.

In 1977 the SOL-20 seemed particularly suited for
student use because of its physical compactness and hardware
flexibility. The motherboard comes with the microprocessor,
video interfacing and memory buffer, ROM monitor, audio tape
interface, and serial and parallel outputs to drive printers and
plotters. The keyboard has upper and lower case letters and
cursor controls convenient for editing manuscripts. The screen
has 16 lines of 64 characters. There is room for five S-100
cards inside of the keyboard console. The author uses one of
these for the disk controller, two for 48K of memory, one for a
numerical processor interface board, and one for a
high-resolution graphics board. The details for the latter two
items are given in the previous chapter.

Such a configuration gives considerable computation
power in a compact package. However, the author has found that
once he had developed the software for his system that it was
not easily transportable to other S-100 bus computers using
other disk hardware and operating systems. The very nature of
the diversity offered by the connector compatability between
products from different manufacturers still tends to limit
distribution of software.

| REFERENCES |
| --- |

If a person purchases one of the more popular microcomputers he/she would be wise to subscribe to one or more of the newsletters or magazines devoted to that particular model. These contain articles and letters written by other users and provide programming tricks, examples, and product evaluations which are not available in the manufacturer's manuals.

CALL A.P.P.L.E.
Apple Pugetsound Program Library Exchange
8710 Salty Drive NW
Olympia, WA 98502

MICRO
(The magazine for 6502 systems)
MICRO INK, Inc.
P. O. Box 6502
Chelmsford, MA 01824

PROG/80
(TRS-80 Programming)
Softside Publications
Milford, NH 03055

PROTEUS / NEWS
(SOL Users Group)
1690 Woodside Road
Redwood City, CA 94061

80-U. S.
(The Journal for TRS-80 Users)
80-NW Publishing
P. O. Box 7112
Tacoma, WA 98407

Chapter 6

COMPARTMENTAL KINETICS:  A FIRST EXAMPLE

The first simulation is a simple one.  It uses the analogy between the volume of a fluid in a leaky tank and the concentration of a substance in a body compartment.  In the simplest case these variables will decay at a rate proportional to how much remains, a situation described by a first-order differential equation.  The solution to this equation is an exponential characterized by an initial value and a rate constant parameter indicating the speed of the decay.  If material is added to the compartment at a constant rate the concentration will reach a steady state at the value which provides an efflux in balance with the influx.

If material is transferred from one leaky compartment to another the concentration in the second will rise to a maximum value and then decay.  Simple as this model is, it provides an analog for comparison with situations in the body in which material may be absorbed by a first-order process and then is lost or metabolized by another such process.  Though the model may not be precise it is useful for conceptualization purposes.

This chapter uses such a model as a starting point, showing how the differential equations are solved digitally. Also included are illustrative displays photographed from the CRT of a microcomputer which has graphic resolution suited for this purpose.  The Chapter Appendix contains a listing of the

James E. Randall, Microcomputers and Physiological Simulation

complete BASIC program which provides the computed responses
shown in the figures.

THE HYDRAULIC MODEL

        Figure 6.1 shows the components of the leaky tank model.
The top tank has a volume A and a leak measured by the parameter
K1.  It empties into the second tank B which also  has  a  leak,
but with a different size of hole, measured by the rate constant
K2.  The problem is to know how much is in the two tanks at  any
time starting with initial values of A and of B and known values
of K1 and K2.  The illustration is an instantaneous view  of  an
animated simulation in which A started with 100 volume units and
B with 0 units.  The shaded area of A  falls  according  to  how
much  remains  in  A  and the area of B initially rises and then
falls.

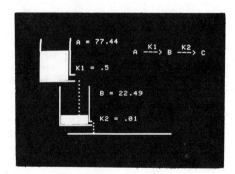

Fig.  6.1.  Instantaneous view
of an animated  simulation  of
the kinetics of two successive
compartments.  The upper  tank
started with  100  units  and
loses material at  a  rate  of
0.5/hour.  As the material in
B accumulates it is lost at  a
rate of 0.01/hr.

        This simple problem can be solved analytically  but  the
point  of  this  chapter  is  to  introduce the topic of graphic
instructional   simulations   in   which   the   student   can
experimentally  test individually the effects of each parameter.
Such an activity develops insight about the role of the two rate
constants,  K1 and  K2,  in  determining the time course of the
amount of material in compartment B.   For  example,  the  peak
value  of  B  is dependent upon the relative values of K1 and K2
while their absolute values determine the time and  duration  of
the  peak.   Such  conclusions  can  be  drawn  from analytical
solutions of the differential equations but graphic displays are
particularly convincing and apt to be remembered.

        This model contains the essence of  many  physiological
processes.  Quantity B can be considered to represent the plasma
concentration of a material which might be absorbed according to
first-order  kinetics and excreted by the same kind  of kinetics

with a different time constant. More realistic considerations
would include factors such as absorption rates limited by a
transport process and an excretion process with a threshold
which had to be exceeded. The model for extracellular glucose,
described in the next chapter, contains some of these
nonlinearities.

```
┌─────────────────────────┐
│  COMPUTED RESPONSES      │
└─────────────────────────┘
```

        The use of this simulation of compartmental kinetics
consists of selecting the initial volumes of A and of B and
setting the rate constants K1 and K2. Many microcomputers have
graphic capabilities which can plot the variables A and B as a
function of time, superimposing successive runs for comparison.
Tabular solutions give more precision but lack visual impact.
The illustrations in this chapter are photographs from the Apple
II microcomputer which has 24 lines of 40 alphanumeric
characters and a high-resolution graphics capability of either
160 or 192 vertical dots by 280 horizontal ones. The
superpositioning of text onto the graphics is done with a
software subroutine read from disk along with the BASIC program.

        Figure 6.2A illustrates the entering of the parameters
and initial conditions for a given run. The program puts in the
title along with any operating instructions (as for correcting
erroneous entries). In the figure the first parameter is
selected as 0.5/hour. Students have to be reminded that the
first-order process is not losing material at a constant
amount/hour, otherwise they may project that 50% will be gone in
1 hour and 100% in 2 hours. Alternative methods of
characterizing first-order processes are presented to the viewer
as soon as K1 is fixed. These include the time constant, the
reciprocal of the rate constant; and the half-life, 0.693 times
the time constant.

        In Figure 6.2A the rate constant for the second
compartment is 0.25/hr and the initial value of A = 1. The
initial value of B is set to zero in the bottom line and the
program is waiting for a RETURN key to be pressed in order to
continue with the solution.

        Figure 6.2B shows the complete graphic solution, a
process which takes 20 seconds to compute and plot. The
ordinate scale is normalized according to the initial value of
A. The exponential fall of A is down to 37% at its time
constant of 2 hours. The initial rate of rise of B matches the
decay in A but as B accumulates the second compartment begins to
lose material according to the value of K2. At 10 hours there
still is some volume left in B.

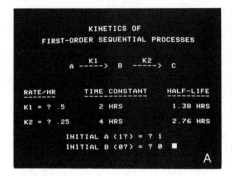
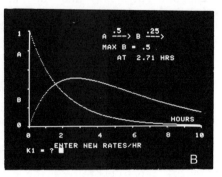

Fig. 6.2. Photographs of the CRT displays for the sequential
compartments simulation. In A the parameters for the two
rate constants are selected and the initial values of the
variables set. In B there is the corresponding computed
solution along with a display indicating the peak value of
the variable B and the time of its occurance. The
variables are normalized to the initial value of A.


        The upper right portion of the display exhibits the rate
constants during the simulation. At the conclusion of the run
there is a display of the maximum value of B and the time at
which it occurs. Note that the display of B has a finite
resolution and that there appears to be a plateau centered at 3
hours, not at the indicated time of the maximum which is at 2.71
hours. This apparent contradiction is resolved when it is
realized that B rises faster than it subseqently falls so that
the peak in B occurs sooner than the center of the plateau on
the display.

        The bottom four lines of the graphic display are
available for text. In Figure 6.2B these are used to ask for
new values of the parameters K1 and K2 for solutions to be
superimposed upon the same display. As the program is written
pressing the RETURN key without any parameter entry will restart
the program.

        Figure 6.3 displays a total of three simulations with
the same rate constant K1 = 0.5/hr but with different values of
K2. The middle curve has K2 = 0.25/hr as before but the other
two show the effects upon B with K2 = 0.7 and with K2 = 0.15.
Note that all three tracings start the same because the initial
change in B is dominated by the entry from A. In the bottom
tracing, in which K2 = 0.7/hr, the material leaves faster than
in the others so that B reaches its peak sooner. The upper

corner of the display shows the maximum value of B and the   time
of its peak for the last set of parameters used.

Fig. 6.3. Solutions with three
different  values of K2 showing
the influence of  changing  the
rate  of  loss upon variable B.
In increasing order of the peak
of  B the values of K2 are 0.7,
0.25, 0.15/hr, respectively.

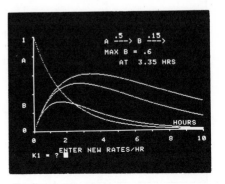

        In principle it is possible to label each curve with its
appropriate rate constant, but this requires  consider  care  to
avoid  overlapping  of  information  and  clutter.   Also it is
possible to identify the individual curves by having them  skip
alternate  points  and  appear  as  dashed  or  dotted  lines.
Microcomputers with color displays also can be used  effectively
for curve identification.

---

THE BASIC PROGRAM

        The  Chapter Appendix contains a complete listing of the
Applesoft  BASIC  program  used  to  generate  the   simulation
exercises  of  the  figures  of  this chapter.  For clarity the
present discussion is limited to the key steps only.  Since this
is  the  first example of simulation, special emphasis is placed
upon the digital integration method and the graphic  display  of
the solutions.  The details of plotting axes, labels, and titles
are omitted at this point.

        The  total  program  is  controlled  by  a  series  of
subroutine calls given in Table 6.1.   This  format  simplifies
discussion and also permits modification for different models of
microcomputers and different versions of BASIC.  The  subroutine
at  line  2500,  called  in  line 110 of the table, displays the
title  and  requests  the  parameters  to  be  used  during  the
simulation.    The  subroutines  at lines 2000 and 5000 draw the
axes, tics, and labels for the graphs.  The main computation and
plotting  statements  are  in the subroutine at line 1000.  Upon
completion of this cycle of events the  program  waits  for  new
values  of the parameters to be entered before going to line 140
to superimpose another solution on the display.

---

Table 6.1

The loop which calls the individual subroutines.    See
the Chapter Appendix for the complete listing.

```
100 REM     MAIN CONTROL LOOP
110 GOSUB 2500                  (Title/parameters
120 HGR                         (Graphics mode
130 GOSUB 2000                  (Axes and tics
140 GOSUB 5000                  (Put K's on graph
150 GOSUB 1000                  (Compute/plot
160 GOSUB 6000                  (New K's
170 GOTO 140                    (New tracing
```

---

The essential features of the subroutine at line 2500
are to request the values of the rate constants, K1 and K2,  and
to request the initial values of the variables A and B. This can
be done by the following four input statements,

```
3030 INPUT "K1 = ";K1
3090 INPUT "K2 = ";K2
3160 INPUT "INIT. A ";A0
3200 INPUT "INIT. B ";B0
3220 DT=10/250: BM=0: TM=0
3230 RETURN
```

The  actual  program  has a method to allow common values of the
parameters to be entered  by  default  simply  by  pressing  the
RETURN  key.   This topic is discussed in later chapters.  Line
3220 in the table sets the computing increment to  10/250  hours
and  sets  two variables which are used in detecting the maximum
value of B and the time of its occurance.

The  simulation  itself  is  performed  by a sequence of
statements given in Table 6.2.  This part of the program  starts
with  the initial values of A and of B and then for 250 steps of
time computes the amount of material  which  enters  and  leaves
these  compartments  during  the  increment  DT.  Preceding each
computation the current values of A and B are plotted using  the
high-resolution  graphics  mode.   Line  1020  contains the FOR
statement with I as the index.

Lines  1030  and 1040 plot the current values of A and B
normalized to A0, the initial value of A.  This uses  the  HPLOT
X,Y  command in which the origin for X=0 and Y=0 is at the upper
left-hand corner of the screen.  Of the total of 280  horizontal
points  on the Apple II screen the first 25 are used for labels.
The ordinates are scaled to fill the 150 vertical  lines  on the

high-resolution screen and the bottom of the screen is used for
4 lines of alphanumeric text. The 250 increments of time
encompass a total of 10 hours for the solutions.

```
                        Table 6.2

    An abbreviated form of the plotting and computation
    subroutine.  See the Chapter Appendix for the complete
    listing.

    1000 REM  DISPLAY AND COMPUTATION
    1010 A=A0: B=B0                    (Initial values
    1020 FOR I=0 TO 250
    1030   HPLOT 25+I,150*(1-A/A0)     (Plot A
    1040   HPLOT 25+I,150*(1-B/B0)     (Plot B
    1050   DA=-K1*A*DT                 (Change in A
    1060   DB=+K1*A*DT -K2*B*DT        (Change in B
    1070   A=A+DA: B=B+DB              (Update A,B
    1090   IF B>BM THEN BM=B:TM=I*DT   (Max B?
    1100   NEXT I
    1180 RETURN
```

The defining equations for the net rate of change of
variables A and B consist of terms related to the gains and
losses of each.  For example,

| Net | Loss | Gain |
|---|---|---|
| $dA/dt$ = | $-K1 * A$ | |
| $dB/dt$ = | $-K2 * B$ | $+K1 * A$ |

By the definition of a first-order process, the loss from each
compartment is directly proportional to the amount which remains
in each.  For compartment B the gain equals the loss from A.

The method used here to find a solution is the simple
Euler rectangular integration in which the rates of change are
assumed to be constant during the computation interval.  There
are more elaborate techniques which do not depend upon this
assumption but if the time increments are small relative to the
time constants involved the accuracy is sufficient for teaching
uses.  The more accurate methods generally take considerably
longer and their complexity may obscure the objectives of an
introductory text such as this.

Lines 1050 and 1060 contain the digital approximations
to changes in A and in B during the increment DT.  Line 1070

uses the computed values of DA and DB to obtain the new values of A and of B which are used on the next iteration. Line 1090 compares the current value of B with the maximum value so far and replaces BM if appropriate. After the total of 250 computations the maximum value of B and the time of its occurance are displayed. The program then waits for a new set of rate constant parameters. As written, the program restarts from the beginning if the RETURN key is pressed without entering any numerical values.

In spite of the possible errors of assuming a constant rate of change over finite time increments, appreciation of the role of lines 1050 and 1060 is important in understanding the idea of digital simulation of physiological systems. Illustration of the simplicity of this operation is the primary purpose of the present chapter. Complexities arise from having more variables which interact with one another, from having nonlinearities of many kinds, and from the additional steps used in more accurate methods of integration. The next chapter considers a slightly more complicated physiological situation in which the concentration of glucose is evaluated in terms of the methods of gaining and losing this substance from the extracellular compartment.

## REFERENCES

Cassano, W. F.: A biological simulation system. Comput. Biomed. Res. 10:383-392 (1977).

Estreicher, J., C. Revillard, and J. Scherrer: Compartmental analysis - I: LINDE, a program using an analytical method of integration with constituent matrices. Comput. biol. Med. 9:49-65 (1979).

Garfinkel, D., C. B. Marback, and N. Z. Shapiro: Stiff differential equations. Ann. Rev. Biophys. Bioeng. 6:525-542 (1977).

## CHAPTER APPENDIX

The following pages contain the complete Applesoft BASIC listing of the program used for the simulations in this chapter. Lines 30-45 load a binary routine from disk which is used to place alphanumerical characters onto the high-resolution graphics screen. The BASIC subroutine which switches from the normal text handler to the graphics version is at line 9000.

```
10   REM     SEQUENTIAL COMPARTMENTS
15   REM     APPLE II GRAPHIC PLOT OF AMOUNT IN TWO LEAKY TANKS
20   REM     SELECT RATE CONSTANTS, INITIAL AMOUNTS
21 :
22 :
25 :
30   REM     LOAD CHARACTER ROUTINE & TABLE
35 D$ =  CHR$ (4):
40   PRINT D$;"BLOAD HI-RES CHARACTER GEN $6000"
45   PRINT D$;"BLOAD CHARACTER TABLE $6800"
50 :
60 :
70 :
100   REM   ---MAIN PROGRAM LOOP---
105   TEXT : HOME : REM   CLEAR SCREEN
110   GOSUB 2500: REM   TITLE/PARAMETERS
120   HOME : HGR : REM   GRAPHICS MODE
130   GOSUB 2000: REM   AXES/TICS
140   GOSUB 5000: REM   PUT K´S ON REACTION <------
150   GOSUB 1000: REM   COMPUTE/PLOT
160   GOSUB 6000: REM   NEW K´S=?
170   GOTO 140: REM   SUPERIMPOSE NEW TRACING --->
180 :
190 :
200 :
1000   REM   ---DISPLAY AND COMPUTE LOOP---
1010 A = A0:B = B0
1020   FOR I = 0 TO 250
1030   HPLOT 25 + I,150 * (1 - A / A0)
1040   HPLOT 25 + I,150 * (1 - B / A0)
1050 DA =  - K1 * A * DT
1060 DB =  + K1 * A * DT - K2 * B * DT
1070 A = A + DA
1080 B = B + DB
1090   IF B > BM THEN BM = B:TM = I * DT
1100   NEXT I
1110   REM   DISPLAY BMAX AND ITS TIME
1120   VTAB 4: HTAB 20
1130 A$ = "MAX B = " +  STR$ ( INT (BM * 100) / 100)
1140   GOSUB 9000: REM   PUT A$ ON HI-RES GRAPH AREA
1150   VTAB 6: HTAB 23
1160 A$ = "AT  " +  STR$ ( INT (100 * TM) / 100) + " HRS"
1170   GOSUB 9000
1180   RETURN
1190 :
1200 :
```

```
2000   REM   ---INITIALIZE SCREEN DISPLAY---
2010   REM   PLOT AXES
2020   HPLOT 25,0 TO 25,150 TO 275,150
2030   FOR I = 0 TO 5
2040   : HPLOT 23,30 * I
2045   : HPLOT 24,30 * I
2050   : NEXT I
2060   FOR I = 0 TO 10
2070   : HPLOT 25 + (I * 25),151
2080   : HPLOT 25 + (I * 25),152
2090   : NEXT I
2100   VTAB 21
2110   PRINT "   0        2        4        6        8        10"
2120   A$ = "A ---> B --->"
2130   VTAB 2: HTAB 20: GOSUB 9000
2140   VTAB 1: HTAB 1:A$ = " 1": GOSUB 9000
2150   VTAB 5: HTAB 2:A$ = "A": GOSUB 9000
2160   VTAB 14: HTAB 2:A$ = "B": GOSUB 9000
2170   VTAB 19: HTAB 2:A$ = "0": GOSUB 9000
2180   VTAB 18: HTAB 34
2190   A$ = "HOURS": GOSUB 9000
2390   RETURN
2400   :
2410   :
2420   :
2500   REM    TEXT ONTO SCREEN; GET PARAMETERS
2520   TEXT : HOME
2530   HTAB 15: PRINT "KINETICS OF "
2540   PRINT : HTAB 5
2550   PRINT "FIRST-ORDER SEQUENTIAL PROCESSES"
2560   VTAB 7: HTAB 15
2570   PRINT "K1          K2"
2580   HTAB 11
2590   PRINT "A -----> B -----> C"
2600   VTAB 13
2610   PRINT "RATE/HR       TIME CONSTANT      HALF-LIFE"
2620   PRINT "-------       -------------      ---------"
2630   PRINT
2640   :
```

```
3000   REM     --GET PARAMETERS--
3010 DT = 10 / 250
3020   HTAB 1: VTAB 16
3030   INPUT "K1 = ? ";K1
3040   HTAB 17: VTAB 16
3050   PRINT  INT (100 / K1) / 100;" HRS";
3060   HTAB 32
3070   PRINT  INT (69 / K1) / 100;" HRS"
3080   HTAB 1: VTAB 19
3090   INPUT "K2 = ? ";K2
3100   HTAB 17: VTAB 19
3110   PRINT  INT (100 / K2) / 100;" HRS";
3120   HTAB 32
3130   PRINT  INT (69 / K2) / 100;" HRS";
3140   HTAB 10: VTAB 22
3150 A0 = 1
3160   INPUT "INITIAL A (1?) = ? ";A$
3170   IF A$ <  > "" THEN A0 =  VAL (A$)
3180 B0 = 0
3190   HTAB 10: VTAB 24
3200   INPUT "INITIAL B (0?) = ? ";A$
3210   IF A$ <  > "" THEN B0 =  VAL (A$)
3220 TM = 0:BM = B0
3230   RETURN
3240 :
3250 :
3260 :
5000   REM  -- PRINT K´S IN UPPER RIGHT --
5020   VTAB 1: HTAB 22
5030 A$ =  STR$ (K1) + "   ": GOSUB 9000
5040   VTAB 1: HTAB 29
5050 A$ =  STR$ (K2) + "   ": GOSUB 9000
5060   VTAB 4: HTAB 20
5070 A$ = "               ": GOSUB 9000
5080   VTAB 6: HTAB 20
5090   GOSUB 9000
5100   RETURN
5110 :
5120 :
```

```
6000   REM : --ASK FOR NEW K´S--
6010   POKE 34,22: REM      TOP OF WINDOW
6020   : HOME : VTAB 24: HTAB 10
6030   PRINT "ENTER NEW RATES/HR";
6040   PRINT
6050   INPUT "   K1 = ? ";A$
6060   IF A$ = "" THEN  GOTO 100: REM  ---->
6070 K1 =  VAL (A$)
6080   VTAB 23: HTAB 15
6090   PRINT "/HR.  HALF-LIFE="; INT (100 * 0.69 / K1) / 100;
6095   PRINT "HRS."
6100   INPUT "   K2 = ? ";A$
6110   IF A$ = "" THEN  GOTO 100: REM  ---->
6120 K2 =  VAL (A$)
6130   VTAB 23: HTAB 15
6140   PRINT "/HR.  HALF-LIFE="; INT (100 * 0.69 / K2) / 100;
6145   PRINT "HRS."
6150 TM = 0:BM = B0
6160   RETURN
6170 :
6180 :
9000   REM   -- PRINT A$ AS HI-RES CHAR --
9010   REM       TRANSFER PRINT OPERATION TO
9020   REM          SUBROUTINE AT PAGE 96 ($6000)
9030 P1 =  PEEK (54):P2 =  PEEK (55)
9040   PR# 0: POKE 54,0: POKE 55,96
9060   PRINT A$;
9070   REM  RESTORE NORMAL PRINT ROUTINE
9080   POKE 54,P1: POKE 55,P2: POKE  - 16301,0
9090   RETURN
```

Chapter 7

THE GLUCOSE TOLERANCE TEST


Simulation of the interaction between plasma glucose and insulin following the infusion of test doses of glucose provides insight about this physiological process. In addition, it illustrates the ease of setting up and solving nonlinear differential equation models for a familiar homeostatic mechanism.

The glucose tolerance test is used clinically to evaluate the ability of the pancreas to release insulin in response to a large dose of glucose given either orally or intravenously. The normal pancreas releases enough insulin to lower the plasma glucose within a few hours, sometimes to the point of producing hypoglycemia. The deficiency of insulin release, characteristic of juvenile-onset diabetes, prolongs the fall of glucose for many hours.

Graphic simulations of the time course of the plasma concentrations of these two variables illustrates the transient properties of homeostatic adjustments which may exhibit underdamped oscillations when the loop has sufficient gain. Digital solutions of the differential equations which describe the gains and losses of plasma insulin and glucose are realistic extentions of the linear sequential compartment model of Chapter 6. The nonlinearities include those which arise from the

James E. Randall, Microcomputers and Physiological Simulation

saturation of the renal absorption process at high plasma levels
of glucose and from the controlled loss of glucose which depends
upon the product of the two variables, insulin and glucose.

One  of the first quantitative models of the dynamics of
this interaction was that of Dr.  Victor  Bolie  (1961).   This
analog  computer  simulation  called  attention  to  the analogy
between the insulin-glucose response and that of servomechanisms
which  are  near  critical damping.  Other modelers pursued this
oscillatory  property,  such  as  Gatewood  et  al  (1968),  a
prediction  which  was  confirmed  clinically  when  continuous
on-line glucose analysis became practical.  The  model  in  this
chapter  is  a  BASIC version of the model of Stolwijk and Hardy
(1974) presented as a teaching  illustration  in  the  Thirteenth
Edition of Mountcastle's _Medical_ _Physiology_ textbook.   Their
presentation  in  both analog computer and digital FORTRAN forms
is probably the first inclusion of computer programs in a  major
medical text.

The  organization  of  this  chapter  starts  with  the
assumptions  of the model and gives the BASIC statements for the
critical steps.  This  is  followed  by  computed  responses  for
normal, depressed, and elevated pancreatic sensitivities.  Other
parameters can be manipulated in the model, such as changing the
glucose  utilization  to  mimic  the  maturity-onset diabetes in
which the cells become  refractory  to  insulin.   The  Chapter
Appendix  consists  of  a  listing  of  the  BASIC program which
produces  the  illustrations  on  an  Apple  computer.   Tabular
solutions  can be obtained by substituting an  appropriate  output
subroutine.

---

| THE INSULIN-GLUCOSE INTERACTION MODEL |

The model given here is identical to the  one  presented
by  Stolwijk  and  Hardy  in FORTRAN except that the symbols are
shortened to two letters to fit the BASIC format.  The  operator
can select all parameters arbitrarily, but the version presented
permits  selecting  the  pancreatic  responsiveness  to  plasma
glucose;  insulin-controlled  glucose  utililzation;  and  the
initial  plasma  concentrations  of  glucose  and  insulin.   The
plotted  responses  are  the  plasma concentrations of these two
variables, but renal spillover can be included easily.

Figure  7.1  shows  the  approximations of the gains and
losses of  the  extracellular  insulin  and  glucose  using  the
symbols  defined  in Table 7.1.  The total extracellular glucose
is a product of its concentration and a volume.  The  units  of
the  concentration  variable  G  are not per ml but rather in mg
glucose/100 ml  (mg%)  so that the  volume  factor  is  not  total

extracellular   volume but a capacitance CG, the number of 100 ml
aliquots in the extracellular volume.   The product (G*CG)   gives
the total extracellular glucose in mg at any instant.

---

Table   7.1.

The symbols used in the model and their normal values.
This   is   a   direct   adaptation   of   Table 57-1 in the
reference cited for Stolwijk and Hardy.


| SYMBOLS | PARAMETERS/VARIABLES | NORMAL VALUES | |
|---------|---------------------|--------------|---|
| EX | Extracellular Space | 15,000 | ml |
| CG | Gluc.capacitance=EX/100 | 150 | |
| CI | Insul.capacitance=EX/100 | 150 | |
| Q | Liver release of glucose | 8,400 | mg/hr |
| QT | Glucose infusion rate | 80,000 | mg/hr |
| IN | Infusion, QT or 0 | | |
| DD | First-order glucose loss | 24.7 | mg/hr/mg% |
| GG | Controlled glucose loss | 13.9 | mg/hr/mg%/mU% |
| GK | Renal threshold | 250 | mg% |
| MU | Renal loss rate | 72 | mg/hr/mg% |
| G0 | Pancreas threshold | 51 | mg% |
| BB | Insulin release rate | 14.3 | mU/hr/mg% |
| AA | First-order insulin loss | 76 | mU/hr/mg% |
| G | Extracellular glucose | 81 | mg% |
| I | Extracellular insulin | 5.5 | mU% |
| T | Time | | hours |
| DT | Computation increment | 1/60 | hrs |

---

The model includes two constant inputs of glucose.   The
rate  of   release  by   the liver is assumed to be the constant Q
with a typical value of 8,400 mg/hr.   In more   elaborate   models
this   would   be   a   variable influenced by sympathetic activity,
epinephrine levels, and glucagon.    The   infusion   of   exogenous
glucose   for   the tolerance test is the constant IN which is set
to 80 grams/hr for 0.5 hours to  provide   a   total   dose   of   40
grams.   At other times IN=0.

Three mechanisms are proposed for the loss   of   glucose.
The   loss   in   the   urine   occurs   when the plasma concentration
exceeds the  saturation of the tubular   reabsorption of glucose.

The parameter GK is used as a threshold for this process. This rate of loss is proportional to the amount by which G exceeds GK, thus introducing a nonlinearity in the equations for gains and losses of glucose. The constant of proportionality MU is determined by the glomerular filtration rate which has 7.2 liters/hour as a typical value.

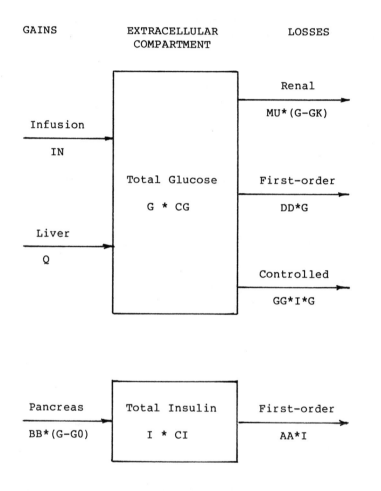

Fig. 7.1. Components of the model for the interaction between glucose and insulin. These molecules are considered as distributed uniformally within the extracellular compartment with approximated mechanisms of increases and losses using parameters defined in Table 7.1. The interaction arises because glucose controls insulin release and insulin controls glucose utilization.

The second loss of extracellular glucose is that which enters cells without insulin. This is considered as a first-order loss based on an assumption that the freely exchangeable concentration of intracellular glucose is negligible. The authors of the model point out that this assumption would not be necessary if there were data about the release of intracellular glucose by glucagon and epinephrine in the hypoglycemic state. The rate constant for this process, DD, is assigned a value of 24.7 mg/hr/mg%, corresponding to a half-life of about 4.2 hours for this mode of disappearance.

The final term in the equation involving glucose rates is a second source of nonlinearity. The loss controlled by insulin is considered to be the product of the two variables, insulin and glucose, and a parameter GG. This factor is a measure of the controlled glucose utilization rate. The clinical condition of maturity-onset diabetes, in which the cellular utilization of glucose becomes refractory to insulin, can be simulated by varying the values of GG from the normal presented in Table 7.1.

The plasma insulin level, expressed in milliunits/100 ml, is considered to have a single input and a single output. The pancreatic release of insulin is determined by the amount the plasma glucose exceeds some threshold G0. In the model this threshold was taken as 51 mg% so that there would be no insulin gain in this hypoglycemic state, another limitation of the simulation. The constant of proportionality for the insulin release, BB, is varied to mimic changes in the pancreatic sensitivity characteristic of juvenile-onset diabetes. The destruction of plasma insulin is considered to be directly proportional to its concentration with a constant of AA. For AA = 76 mU/hr/mg%, the value used, the half-life is 1.4 hours.

```
THE BASIC PROGRAM
```

This section discusses the major steps involved in the simulation program, using the symbols defined in Table 7.1 and the gains and losses defined in Figure 7.1. The Chapter Appendix contains the complete listing for the program written in Applesoft BASIC for graphic display of the computed variables.

Table 7.2 gives the initialization steps (lines 110 and 120) and the main computation loop (lines 1000–1080). Initialization consists of setting the computation parameters and then plotting the axes and labels. Table 7.3 gives the essential steps of the subroutine at line 5000 which sets the parameters to the values given in Table 7.1. Any or all of

these  can be chosen by the operator but the suggested option is
to be able to set the pancreatic sensitivity (BB) to some  value
normalized  to  the  baseline  value  of  14.3.  In addition the
normalized  glucose utilization  factor  (GG)  is  selectable  in
order  to  simulate the maturity-onset diabetes.  Initial values
of glucose (G) and of insulin (I) are  selectable  in  order  to
start  the  simulation from their respective steady-state levels
appropriate  for  the  chosen  pancreatic  gain  and  glucose
utilization coefficient.

---

Table 7.2

The major steps  in  the  model  for  the  interaction
between  glucose  and  insulin.  After  the  model's
parameters are chosen and the axes  plotted  the  main
program  plots  251  values  of glucose and of insulin
concentration as computed at one-minute intervals.

```
100 REM                    (Initialization
110 GOSUB 5000             (Get parameters
120 GOSUB 4000             (Axes and labels
130:
1000 REM                   (Main program
1010 FOR K=0 to 250        (Counts plotted points
1020     FOR J=1 to 2      (Computations/plotted point
1030     GOSUB 3000        (Compute variables
1040     T = T + DT        (Increment time
1050     NEXT J            (Another computation
1060 GOSUB 2000            (Plot variables
1070 NEXT K                (Again
1080 GET A$: GOTO 100      (Press any key to restart
```

---

The  subroutine  at  line 4000, which plots the axes and
places the insulin and glucose scales on the  ordinate  and  the
hours  on  the  abcissa, is not discussed here since the details
depend upon whether graphic or tabular output displays are being
used  and  also can vary with the type of computer.  The version
for te Apple  II  computer,  using  a  software  high-resolution
character  generator  on  the  graph,  is  listed  in lines 4000
through 4450 of the Chapter Appendix.

The  main  program at lines 1000-1080 of Table 7.2 plots
251  points  on  the  graph  at  increments  of  two times the
computation  increment  of  DT=1/60 hour.  This simulation of a
total time of eight hours executes in 60 seconds.

```
                        Table 7.3

An  abbreviated  form of the subroutine which sets the
parameters for the simulation.  The operator picks the
glucose    utilization,   pancreatic   sensitivity,   and
initial concentrations of glucose  and  insulin.   The
complete  listing is in lines 5000-5390 of the Chapter
Appendix.

5000 REM                          (Get parameters
5010 T=0: DT=1/60                 (Time in hours
5080 T1=1: T2=1.5                 (Start,stop in
5130 EX=15000:CG=EX/100:CI=EX/100 (Excell volume
5150 Q=8400: QT=80000             (Glucose inputs
5180 DD=24.7:GG=13.9:GK=250:MU=72 (Glu output
5200 INPUT "GLU UTIL ?";GG        (Controlled loss
5250 G0=51:AA=76                  (Insulin param.
5270 INPUT "PANCREAS ?";BB        (Release
5340 INPUT "INIT I ?";I           (Initial insulin
5370 INPUT "INIT G ?";G           (Initial glucose
5390 RETURN
```

The computation subroutine  starting  at  line  3000  is
listed  in  detail  in  Table  7.4.  Lines 3020 and 3030 set the
infusion rate IN to the value QT (80  grams/hour)  if  the  time
variable  T  is  between T1 and T2, otherwise IN = 0.  Line 3040
calculates  the  change  in  total  glucose  mass  during  the
integration  interval  of  DT=1/60  hour.  These changes include
liver release (Q), infusion (IN), controlled loss (GG*I*G),  and
first-order  loss  (DD*G).   Line 3050 subtracts the renal loss
(MU*(G-GK)) if concentration G exceeds the threshold GK.   Note
that  the  individual  gains  and losses are in milligrams/hour.
Line 3060 updates the glucose in units of mg/100 ml.

Lines  3070-3100  of  Table  7.4 calculate the change in
insulin concentration during the one-minute interval.  Line 3080
has  the  first-order loss (AA*I).  Line 3090 has the pancreatic
release (BB*(G-G0)) provided that G exceeds  the  threshold  G0.
Line 3100 updates the insulin in milliunits/100 ml.

The  subroutine  at  line  2000  plots  the  computed
concentrations  on  the  previously  plotted axes.  The complete
listing for an Apple  II  graphic  display  is  given  in  lines
2000-2090  with  the  insulin curve plotted as a broken line for
identification.  For a tabular output this suroutine  should  be
changed  to  one  with printing commands.  After 251 points have
been plotted pressing any key restarts the exercise.

Table 7.4

The computation of glucose and insulin concentration changes during the DT increment. The separate gains and losses are diagrammed in Figure 7.1.

```
3000 REM    GLUCOSE CHANGE DURING DT        (Computations
3020 IN=0                                   (Infusion rate
3030 IF T=>T1 AND T=<T2 THEN IT=QT          (=QT for T1-T2
3040 DG = (Q+IN-(GG*I*G)-DD*G)*DT           (Glucose
3050 IF G=>GK THEN DG=DG-(MU*(G-GK))*DT      (Renal spill
3060 G = G + DG/CG                          (G concen
3070 REM    INSULIN CHANGE DURING DT
3080 DI = (-AA*I) * DT                       (1st-order
3090 IF G=>G0 THEN DI=DI+(BB*(G-G0))*DT     (Pancr release
3100 I = I + DI/CI                          (I concen
3110 RETURN
```

COMPUTED RESPONSES

This section illustrates the glucose and insulin responses for infusion of 40 grams of glucose over a 30-minute period. The parameter which is varied in the different simulations is the coefficient (BB) which indicates the rate of release of insulin as a function of the amount of glucose which exceeds a threshold amount (G0). Alternatively, the program provides the opportunity to manipulate the glucose utilization parameter GG in order to illustrate the clinical condition in which this response is reduced.

Figure 7.2A shows the CRT display by which a student can enter the parameters and initial conditions for the simulation. In the figure the infusion rate of 80 grams/hour is to start at 1 hour and terminate at 1.5 hours. The normalized glucose utilization is set to unity by assigning the value of 13.9 to parameter GG, the coefficient relating glucose disappearance with insulin concentration. Similarly the default value of pancreatic sensitivity is set to one by setting the coefficient BB=14.3. The steady-state values of insulin and glucose for these values of system parameters are 5.5 mU% and 81 mg% respectively.

Figure 7.2B is the CRT display of the simulation with the ordinate showing the glucose and insulin scales. The total simulation is for over 8 hours with the glucose infusion graphed from 1 to 1.5 hours. During this time the glucose increases at an approximately constant rate until the rate is reduced when the concentration exceeds the renal threshold of 250 mg%. Upon the termination of the infusion the glucose is lost by the three different methods as described before.

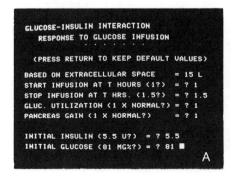
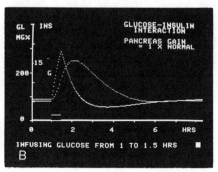

Fig 7.2.   Simulation   of the   normal response   of   glucose and insulin to infusion of glucose. In A the parameters have been selected such that there is normal pancreatic sensitivity and glucose utilization. In B the glucose rise stimulates the release of insulin which in turn lowers glucose levels.

The rise of glucose increases the insulin level which reaches a peak at two hours, later than the glucose maximum. As insulin increase speeds the glucose-controlled loss as this substrate moves into the cells. Note that at 3 to 4 hours the situation is actually hypoglycemic, an undershoot characteristic of many underdamped homestatic mechanisms.

Eventually a steady state is reached once again in which the glucose losses match the 8 grams/hour postulated as being released by the liver. The steady-state value of insulin is that concentration required to have its release from the pancreas match its destruction and still satisfy the interrelatonship with glucose concentration.

Figure 7.3 illustrates the response which occurs if the pancreatic sensitivity is reduced to 0.2 times normal. To avoid a transient the initial concentration of insulin is set to 140 mg% and the insulin to 2.9 mU%, the steady-state values of these variables for the reduced amount of insulin released by the pancreas. Note the reduction in the insulin response and the prolonged glucose level, conditions characteristic of this type of diabetes.

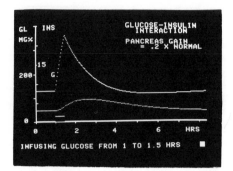

Fig. 7.3. A simulation of the reduced pancreatic sensitivity type of diabetes. The initial values are set to steady-state values as determined by a run with no glucose infusion. The small response of the insulin, the dotted tracing, explains the slower fall as compared to the normal condition.

The display in Figure 7.4 is the case in which the insulin response of the pancreas is exaggerated from normal, as might be the case for a tumerous condition. In this simulation the pancreatic gain is set to two times normal and the steady-state value of insulin is higher and that for glucose is lower than for normal. The exact values can not be found analytically, because of the nonlinearities involved, but they can be found by simulating the condition in which there is no infusion of glucose as by starting and stopping the infusion at the same time.

During infusion the glucose rise is similar to normal but note the large response of the insulin release. It in turn increases the controlled loss of glucose so that the concentration of that material falls below the initial baseline value.

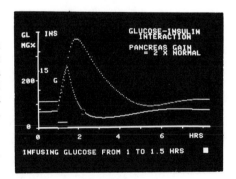

Fig. 7.4. Simulation of an elevated response of pancreas release of insulin to a test dose of glucose. The dotted tracing is that of insulin which has an initial steady-state value of 6.9 mU%. That for glucose is 69.4 mg%.

REFERENCES

Bolie, V. W.: Coefficients of normal blood glucose regulation. J. Appl. Physiol. 16:783-788 (1961).

Gatewood, L. C., E. Ackerman, J. W. Rosevear, G. D. Molnar, and T. W. Burns: Tests of a mathematical model of the blood-glucose regulatory system. Comput. & Biomed. Res. 2:1-14 (1968).

Lafferty, H. H., A. E. B. Giddings, and D. Mangnall: A digital computer model for glucose-insulin dynamics. Comput. Biol. & Med. 8:41-55 (1978).

Stolwijk, J. A. J., and J. D. Hardy: Regulation and control in physiology. Chapter 57 in Medical Physiology, Thirteenth Edition. V. B. Mountcastle, Ed. St. Louis: C. V. Mosby Co. (1974).

CHAPTER APPENDIX

The following pages contain the listing of the insulin-glucose interaction program for Applesoft BASIC. For use with other computers the graphic display subroutines at lines 2000 and 4000 would have to be replaced. For placing labels on the graphs the listed program calls in the character generator subroutine from disk as supplied in Apple Software Bank Contributed Programs Volume 3. It takes approximately one minute to simulate the glucose and insulin responses over a total period of 8 hours.

```
10   REM  --- GLUCOSE TOLERANCE TEST ---
15   REM  MODEL OF STOLWIJK AND HARDY, CHAPTER 57
20   REM   IN 13TH EDITION MOUNTCASTLE'S MEDICAL PHYSIOLOGY
25 :
30 :
35   REM   LOAD BINARY FOR TEXT ON GRAPHS
40 D$ =  CHR$ (4)
45   PRINT D$;"BLOAD HI-RES CHARACTER GEN $6000"
50   PRINT D$;"BLOAD CHARACTER TABLE $6800"
55 :
60 :
100   REM  -- INITIALIZATION --
110   GOSUB 5000: REM   GET PARAMETERS
120   GOSUB 4000: REM   AXES AND LABELS
130 :
140 :
1000   REM  -- MAIN PROGRAM --
1010   FOR K = 0 TO 250: REM      PLOT COUNTER
1020   ::: FOR J = 1 TO 2: REM    COMPUTATIONS/PLOT
1030   ::: GOSUB 3000: REM        COMPUTE VARIABLES
1040   ::::T = T + DT
1050   ::: NEXT J: REM            ANOTHER COMPUTE
1060   :: GOSUB 2000: REM         PLOT VARIABLES
1070   :: NEXT K: REM             ANOTHER
1080   HTAB 39: VTAB 24: GET A$: GOTO 100
1090 :
1100 :
2000   REM  -- PLOT INFUSION, GLUCOSE, INSULIN --
2010 X = 25 + K: REM   ABCISSA
2020 Y = 150 - 1 - (IN / 10000): IF Y < 0 THEN Y = 0
2030   HPLOT X,Y
2040 Y = 150 - G * (150 / 400): IF Y < 0 THEN Y = 0
2050   HPLOT X,Y
2060   IF X / 2 -  INT (X / 2) < .4 THEN 2090
2070 Y = 150 - I * 6: IF Y < 0 THEN Y = 0
2080   HPLOT X,Y
2090   RETURN
2100 :
2110 :
3000   REM   -- COMPUTE NEW GLUCOSE, INSULIN --
3010   REM  GLUCOSE CHANGE DURING DT
3020 IN = 0: REM   INFUSION RATE
3030   IF T = > T1 AND T = < T2 THEN IN = QT
3040 DG = (Q + IN - GG * I * G - DD * G) * DT
3050   IF G = > GK THEN DG = DG - (MU * (G - GK)) * DT: REM   RNL
3060 G = G + DG / CG: REM   CONCENTRATION CHANGE
3070   REM  INSULIN CHANGE DURING DT
3080 DI = ( - AA * I) * DT: REM   FIRST-ORDER LOSS
3090   IF G = > G0 THEN DI = DI + (BB * (G - G0)) * DT: REM   ADD
3100 I = I + DI / CI: REM   CONCENTRATION CHANGE
3110   RETURN
```

```
4000   REM   -- AXES AND LABELS --
4010   HOME : HGR
4020   HPLOT 25,150 TO 275,150
4030   FOR X = 25 TO 275 STEP 30: REM   HOUR TICS
4040   HPLOT X,151 TO X,152: NEXT
4050   HPLOT 25,0 TO 25,150
4060   FOR Y = 0 TO 150 STEP 37.5: REM   GLU TICS
4070   HPLOT 22,Y TO 24,Y: NEXT
4080   FOR Y = 0 TO 150 STEP 30: REM   INS TICS
4090   HPLOT 26,Y TO 28,Y: NEXT
4100   HTAB 24: VTAB 1
4110 A$ = "GLUCOSE-INSULIN": GOSUB 9000
4120   HTAB 26: VTAB 2
4130 A$ = "INTERACTION": GOSUB 9000
4140   HTAB 1: VTAB 24
4150   PRINT "INFUSING GLUCOSE FROM ";
4160   PRINT  INT (10 * T1) / 10;" TO ";
4170   PRINT  INT (10 * T2) / 10;" HRS";
4180   HTAB 1: VTAB 10
4190 A$ = "200": GOSUB 9000
4200   HTAB 2: VTAB 19
4210 A$ = "0": GOSUB 9000
4220   HTAB 1: VTAB 1
4230 A$ = "GL": GOSUB 9000
4240   HTAB 1: VTAB 3
4250 A$ = "MG%": GOSUB 9000
4260   HTAB 5: VTAB 1
4270 A$ = " INS": GOSUB 9000
4280   HTAB 5: VTAB 8
4290 A$ = "15": GOSUB 9000
4300   HTAB 10: VTAB 4
4310 A$ = "G": GOSUB 9000
4320   HTAB 17: VTAB 13
4330 A$ = "I": GOSUB 9000
4340   HTAB 4: VTAB 21: PRINT "0";
4350   HTAB 13: VTAB 21: PRINT "2";
4360   HTAB 21: VTAB 21: PRINT "4";
4370   HTAB 30: VTAB 21: PRINT "6";
4380   HTAB 36: VTAB 21: PRINT "HRS";
4390   HTAB 24: VTAB 4
4400 A$ = "PANCREAS GAIN": GOSUB 9000
4410   HTAB 27: VTAB 5
4420 A$ = "= " +  STR$ (BG) + " X NORMAL": GOSUB 9000
4430   RETURN
4440 :
4450 :
```

```
5000   REM  -- GET PARAMETERS --
5010   TEXT : HOME :T = 0:DT = 1 / 60
5020   PRINT : PRINT "GLUCOSE-INSULIN INTERACTION"
5030   PRINT : PRINT "   RESPONSE TO GLUCOSE INFUSION"
5040   PRINT : PRINT
5050   PRINT "(PRESS RETURN TO KEEP DEFAULT VALUES)"
5060   PRINT : PRINT
5070   PRINT "BASED ON EXTRACELLULAR SPACE    = 15 L"
5080   PRINT :T1 = 1:T2 = 1.5: REM  DEFAULT TIMES
5090   INPUT "START INFUSION AT T HOURS (1?)   = ? ";A$
5100   IF A$ <  > "" THEN T1 =  VAL (A$)
5110   PRINT : INPUT "STOP INFUSION AT T HRS. (1.5?)   = ? ";A$
5120   IF A$ <  > "" THEN T2 =  VAL (A$)
5130 EX = 15000:CG = EX / 100:CI = EX / 100
5140   REM  GLUCOSE GAINS
5150 Q = 8400: REM  LIVER RELEASE=8.4 GRAMS/HR
5160 QT = 80000: REM   INFUSE 80 GRAMS/HOUR
5170   REM  GLUCOSE LOSSES
5180 DD = 24.7: REM  FIRST-ORDER LOSS RATE
5190 GG = 13.9:UT = 1: REM  CONTROLLED UTILIZATION
5200   PRINT : INPUT "GLUC. UTILIZATION (1 X NORMAL?) = ? ";A$
5210   IF A$ <  > "" THEN UT =  VAL (A$):GG = GG * UT
5220 GK = 250: REM  MG % RENAL THRESHOLD
5230 MU = 72: REM  RENAL LOSS RATE
5240   REM  INSULIN GAINS
5250 G0 = 51: REM  MG % PANCREAS GLUCOSE THRESHOLD
5260 BB = 14.3:BG = 1: REM  DEFAULT PANCR GAIN
5270   PRINT : INPUT "PANCREAS GAIN (1 X NORMAL?)    = ? ";A$
5280   IF A$ <  > "" THEN BB = BB *  VAL (A$):BG = BG *  VAL (A$)
5290   REM  INSULIN LOSSES
5300 AA = 76: REM  FIRST-ORDER LOSS RATE
5310   REM   APPROX NORMAL S-S INITAL VALUES
5320   PRINT : PRINT : PRINT
5330 I = 5.5
5340   INPUT "INITIAL INSULIN (5.5 U?)   = ? ";A$
5350   IF A$ <  > "" THEN I =  VAL (A$)
5360 G = 81
5370   PRINT : INPUT "INITIAL GLUCOSE (81 MG%?) = ? ";A$
5380   IF A$ <  > "" THEN G =  VAL (A$)
5390   RETURN
5400 :
5410 :
9000   REM  -- PRINT A$ AS HI-RES CHAR --
9010   REM  BINARY ROUTINE FOR GRAPHICS TEXT
9020 P1 =  PEEK (54):P2 =  PEEK (55)
9030   PR# 0: POKE 54,0: POKE 55,96
9040   PRINT A$;
9050   REM  RETURN NORMAL TEXT PRINTER
9060   POKE 54,P1: POKE 55,P2
9070   POKE  - 16301,0
9080   RETURN
```

Chapter 8

CARDIOVASCULAR SYSTEM MECHANICS


This chapter presents a simplified mechanical model for the cardiovascular system to serve two purposes. First, the author thinks that in spite of the simplifying assumptions used the model contains the essential conceptual framework for appreciation of the strong mechanical coupling between the output from the ventricles and the venous and arterial blood compartments. Such an integrative view can provide the beginning student with a logical basis for understanding how the system works. Then, starting from this vantage point, it is possible to assimilate the many qualitative details which influence the model's fundmental mechanical properties in very complex ways.

The second reason for presenting a cardiovascular model is that because of its physical nature the system is conducive to quantitative formulations and can serve as a good illustration of physiological simulation. The references at the end of the chapter constitute only a small sample of the tremendous amount of work in this area. The model in this chapter is considerably more simplified than most of these but still contains the minimum essentials according to the teaching appoach which the author developed through association with Dr. Fred Grodins at Northwestern University Medical School.

James E. Randall, Microcomputers and Physiological Simulation

The viewpoint, popular with physical scientists who frequently call it a "systems approach", is to characterize each major functional component in the cardiovascular system individually by a mathematical expression arising from experimental observations or approximating assumptions. The behavior of the total system can then be calculated and predicted from the solution which satisfies all component equations simulataneously. These simultaneous equations can be solved by finding the intersections of plotted functions on "ventricular function" and "venous return" curves as used in many physiology textbooks, or by computer simulation.

Before looking at the model in detail let us consider an overall view. This presentation considers only the relationships describing the gross functions of the right and left ventricles and of the total systemic and total pulmonic vascular beds. The relationships are considered to be linear and the physical parameters are rough approximations chosen to provide representative values of the computed variables.

For example, the Starling "Law of the Heart" can be approximated by an expression having cardiac output as the dependent variable and central venous (filling) pressure and arterial (afterload) pressure as independent variables. In the simplified case cardiac output may be considered to vary directly with filling pressure and inversely with afterload pressure with the constant of proportionality being a "contractility" index influenced by such things as myocardial mass, sympathetic activity, and myocardial metabolism.

In the present model the systemic and pulmonic vascular circuits are composed of three compartments each, the arterial and venous compartments having volumes and compliances, and the vascular beds having only resistance as shown in diagramatic form in Figure 8.1. With cardiac output (total circuit blood flow) as the dependent variable the physical equations have arterial and venous pressures as the independent variables and the vascular bed resistance as a constant of proportionality. Besides the pulmonary and peripheral resistances other parameters are the arterial and venous compliances of each major circuit and the total blood volume. These are similar to Otto Frank's classic "windkessel" model for the aorta. The governing relationship for peripheral flow is "Poiseuille's Law" in which flow is directly proportional to arterial-venous pressure gradient and inversely to vascular resistance.

The essence of this point of view is that at any instant the values of these physical parameters (ventricular contractility, blood volume, vascular compliances, and resistances) along with the functional relationships determine the unique solution (cardiac output, arterial and venous pressures, and blood volume distribution) which satisfies all relationships simultaneously.  Pathology and stress upon the cardiovascular system provide new solutions, or "operating points" by modifying one or more of the physical parameters. One important feature of the computer simulations is that they provide an opportunity for students to test the logical consequences of changing one cardiovascular parameter at a time.

For example, the reduction in left ventricular contractility produces a new solution with a significant shift of blood into the pulmonary venous compartment where the elevated filling pressure assists in maintaining cardiac output, as in congestive failure.  Also, an increase in myocardial contractility (hypertrophy) is required to maintain normal cardiac output in the face of the elevated peripheral resistance characteristic of essential hypertension.

The simulation consists of formulating the relationships in the computer language BASIC and assigning typical values for the parameters.  Steady-state solutions use expressions for the variables in terms of the given parameters.  Transient solutions, such as those describing the redistribution of blood following a sudden hemorrhage of the venous volume, involve repeating updates of aortic volume as blood enters from the ventricle at one rate and leaves through the systemic bed at the other end until the two rates are equal in the steady state.

These temporal simulations are slower than the changes observed in real life because the model lacks the fast-responding neural influences which modify parameters such as heart rate, venous compliance, peripheral resistance, and ventricular contractility.  Since the graphic solutions for the linear differential equations will be first-order exponentials the simulations presented here use only tabular solutions and thus emphasize the numerical values of pressures, volume distribution, and cardiac outputs for different physiological conditions.  This also means that these simulations require no special hardware enhancements and should run on any computer equipped with BASIC.

---

## THE FUNCTIONAL RELATIONSHIPS

Figure 8.1 illustrates the arrangement of the major mechanical parameters associated with the model used in this chapter.  Cardiac function is reduced to a left and a right ventricle which can be characterized by contractility coefficients, $K(1)$ and $K(2)$ respectively.  The systemic vascular beds are lumped into compartments having an arterial compliance $AC(1)$, a venous compliance $VC(1)$, and the systemic peripheral resistance $R(1)$.  Similarly the pulmonic circuit is considered

to consist of arterial and venous compartments, with compliances
of AC(2) and VC(2), and a pulmonic resistance R(2).   The total
blood  volume  BV  is  distributed among the arterial and venous
compartments depending upon the values of the other parameters.

     The  tabulation in Table 8.1 gives representative values
for each of these constants, the exact magnitudes  being  chosen
to  give  representative  computed  variables  in  physiological
ranges.   In living systems these properties are not constant but
are  influenced  by  neural  and  humeral  factors  and are also
functions of their associated  variables.    For  instance,  the
arterial  vascular  compliance  is less at high pressure and with
sympathetic activity.  Nevertheless, the user of  such  a  model
should  note  that  the  relative  values of arterial and venous
compliances and the differences between  systemic  and  pulmonic
resistances  for  these  differences  are  responsible  for  the
distribution of blood volume and the pressures.

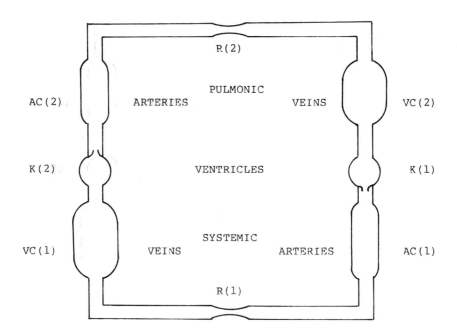

Fig. 8.1.  The components of the mechanical model.  The systemic
      and  pulmonic  vascular  circuits  are  each  lumped  into
      arterial  and  venous  compartments  having  constant
      compliances  and  a  component  exhibiting only resistance.
      The  total  blood  volume  (BV)  is  distributed  among  the
      vascular compartments.

```
Table 8.1

The parameters of the cardiovascular model.  The index
(1)  applies to the systemic vascular components; (2),
to the pulmonary circuit.  The approximations are   not
from   experimental   data   but their relative values do
provide   reasonable   system   pressures,   volumes   and
outputs for teaching purposes.


        PHYSICAL PARAMETERS                APPROXIMATIONS

  K(1)  L. ventr. contractility      1,000 ml/min/mm Hg
  K(2)  R. ventr. contractility      1,000 ml/min/mm Hg

  AC(1) Syst. art. compliance          4.0 ml/mm Hg
  AC(2) Pulm. art. compliance          1.5 ml/mm Hg
  VC(1) Syst. ven. compliance          700 ml/mm Hg
  VC(2) Pulm. ven. compliance          300 ml/mm Hg

  R(1)  Systemic   resistance        0.018 mm Hg/ml/min
  R(2)  Pulmonic   resistance        0.002 mm Hg/ml/min

  BV    Total blood volume           5,500 ml
```

Figure 8.2 and Table 8.2 identify the computed variables
in the model.  These include   the   left   and   right  ventricular
outputs,   CO(1)   and   CO(2),   respectively.  The systemic circuit
contains the arterial volume AV(1), the arterial pressure AP(1),
the   venous   volume   VV(1),   and the venous pressure VP(1).   The
pulmonic   circuit   contains   similar   variables   denoted   with   the
index   (2).     Since   flows   may   not necessarily be equal to one
another or to cardiac output these are defined as FL(1) for   the
peripheral   runoff   and FL(2) for pulmonary flow.  The values for
the variables in Table 8.2 are those that   would   apply   in   the
steady state for the parameters given in Table 8.1.

Table 8.3 contains the functional relationships for   the
components in this model.  The Starling observations obtained in
the isolated heart-lung   preparation   demonstrated   that   stroke
work   is   a   function of end-diastolic volume.  With   simplifying
assumptions the venous filling pressure can be considered as   an
index   of   end-diastolic volume and the stroke work a product of
stroke volume and mean arterial pressure.    Thus   for   a   given
heart   rate one would expect the cardiac output to increase with
greater   venous   filling   pressure   and   decrease   with   greater
arterial   pressures   as long as the heart was functioning on the
compensating or ascending limb of the classic Starling curve.

In the formulations used here this relationship is expressed (in BASIC notation) as:

CO(1) = K(1) * VP(2) - 0.01 * K(1) * [AP(1) - 100].

The first right-hand factor says that left ventricular output is directly proportional to pulmonary venous pressure as long as the systemic arterial pressure is equal to 100. The contractility K(1) is the slope of the left ventricular function curve but does not include the more realistic "decompensated" region where the myocardium is overextended. Its numerical value is increased with sympathetic activity.

The second factor includes the afterloading effect which arterial pressure has upon stroke volume and cardiac output. More extensive models are required for greater realism in regard to both of these components which influence cardiac output but the lesson for the beginning student is to realize that this variable is much more sensitive to changes in venous filling pressure than it is to changes in arterial afterloads.

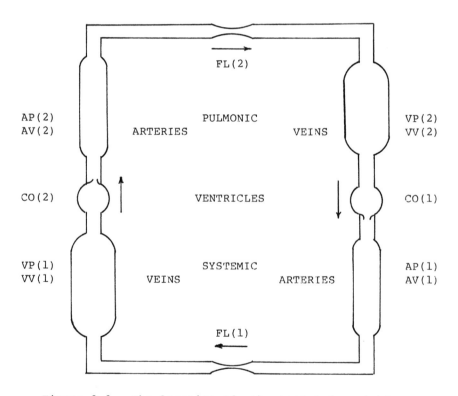

Figure 8.2.  The location of  the computed variables.

Table 8.2

Computed variables in the model. The steady-state values are those which simultaneously satisfy the functional relationships for all individual components when the parameters are are those of Table 8.1.

| COMPUTED VARIABLES | | | STEADY-STATE VALUES | |
|---|---|---|---|---|
| CO(1) | Left ventricular output | | 5,097 | ml/min |
| CO(2) | Right ventricular output | | 5,097 | ml/min |
| | | | | |
| AP(1) | Systemic arterial pressure | | 97 | mm Hg |
| AP(2) | Pulmonic arterial pressure | | 15 | mm Hg |
| VP(1) | Systemic venous pressure | | 5 | mm Hg |
| VP(2) | Pulmonic venous pressure | | 5 | mm Hg |
| | | | | |
| AV(1) | Systemic arterial volume | | 387 | ml |
| AV(2) | Pulmonic arterial volume | | 23 | ml |
| VV(1) | Systemic venous volume | | 3,570 | ml |
| VV(2) | Pulmonic venous volume | | 1,520 | ml |
| | | | | |
| FL(1) | Systemic circuit bloodflow | | 5,097 | ml/min |
| FL(2) | Pulmonic circuit bloodflow | | 5,097 | ml/min |

The pressures in the vascular compartments are considered to be directly proportional to their volumes with compliances as a reciprocal constant, or P=V/C. This, of course, is full of simplifying assumptions but the importance of compliances and their relative values are the lessons being stressed in this exercise, not the exact curvature of pressure versus volume functions. The sum of the four compartmental volumes is the total blood volume BV.

The flow through each of the two vascular circuits is considered to be directly proportional to the respective arterial-venous pressure gradients and inversely to the corresponding resistances. For the systemic flow this would be

$$FL(1) = [AP(1) - VP(1)] / R(1)$$

with a similar expression for the pulmonic side except that (2) is the index.

Microcomputers have the computational capacity to include refinements on this elementary model. All that is lacking is realistic formulations and accompanying software.

Possible extensions which have been done previously by
cardiovascular physiologists could include:

   1) Subdividing the total systemic circuit into
regional compartments, so that the vascular
resistances of each could be varied individually.
This could provide insight regarding the distribution
of cardiac output to segments such as the viscera,
kidney, skeletal muscle, skin, coronary, and cerebral
vascular beds.

   2) To incorporate the important property of heart
rate. One way to do this would be to have part of the
blood volume contained within the two ventricles and
to have stroke volume as a function of end-diastolic
volume which in turn would be influenced not only by
venous filling pressure but also by diastolic filling
time.

   3) Include baroreceptor modulation of heart
properties and add a resistance term to the venous
compartment.

---

Table 8.3

Functional relationships for the individual components
in the mechanical model. The system's variables will
satisfy all of these equations simultaneously for
given values of the physical parameters of blood
volume, compliances, resistances and contractilities.
In the steady state the outputs of the two ventricles
and the flows through the two circuits are identical.


CO(1) = K(1) * VP(2) - 0.01 * K(1) * [AP(1) - 100]
CO(2) = K(2) * VP(1) - 0.01 * K(2) * [AP(2) -  15]

AP(1) = AV(1) / AC(1)
AP(2) = AV(2) / AC(2)
VP(1) = VV(1) / VC(1)
VP(2) = VV(2) / VC(2)

 BV   = AV(1) + VV(1) + AV(2) + VV(2)

FL(1) = [AP(1) - VP(1)] / R(1)
FL(2) = [AP(2) - VP(2)] / R(2)

```
┌─────────────────────────────┐
│  STEADY-STATE SOLUTIONS      │
└─────────────────────────────┘
```

        The objective of the simulations for steady-state
conditions is to examine the consequences upon the integrated
system when a single physical parameter is modified.    For
example, what would be the redistribution of total blood volume
when the left ventricular contractility is reduced to 50% of
normal, a condition simulating severe congestive failure?  A
computer program to accomplish this would ask for the physical
parameters indicated in Table 8.1, solve for the variables in
Table 8.2 which would simultaneously satisfy the functional
relationships in Table 8.3, and then display or print those
variables of particular interest in the exercise.  These basic
steps will be discussed as a set of subroutines called from the
following main program:

```
        100 REM    STATIC CV MODEL
        110 GOSUB 2000          (Set normal values of parameters
        120 GOSUB 3000          (Change one or more parameters
        130 GOSUB 1000          (Calculate variables
        140 GOSUB 4000          (Display calculated variables
        150 GOTO 120            (Repeat; last values as default
```

        Line 110 calls a subroutine starting in line 2000 which
sets all parameters to the normal values given in Table 8.1.
The subroutine at line 3000 called in line 120 asks for values
of these parameters one at a time and offers an opportunity to
change one or more of them.  Line 130 calls the subroutine which
solves the simulataneous equations and Line 140 calls the output
display subroutine.  At this point the program starts over, but
using the most recent parameters rather than the normal ones
used initially.   The full routines for accomplishing each of
these operations are too detailed for our purposes but general
comments may be useful to anyone attempting this simulation.


SETTING THE PARAMETERS

        The routines for entering the values of the physical
parameters and for printing or displaying the computed
steady-state variables in the model depend both upon the
specific objectives of the teaching exercise and upon the
version of BASIC being used.  There are two general comments to
be made about the methods of setting the physical properties in
the program within the context of a teaching exercise.  Rather
than expecting anyone to enter all nine parameters identified in
Table 8.1 it is more convenient to have default values initially
for each of the variables and then have the operator be
concerned only with changes from these.

If an INPUT statement query is answered with only a RETURN on the TRS-80 and CP/M versions of Microsoft BASIC the value of the input variable will remain unchanged. Thus for these computers the steps would be to set initial default values and then ask for the parameters one at a time, letting the user respond with a simple RETURN for those which were not to be changed. The following subroutine sets the parameters according to the values given in Table 8.1.

```
2000 REM  SET DEFAULT VALUES OF PARAMETERS
2010 K(1)=1000:   K(2)=1000         (Contractilities
2020 AC(1)=4  :   AC(2)=1.5         (Arter compliances
2030 VC(1)=700:   VC(1)=300         (Venous compliances
2040 R(1)=0.018:  R(2)=0.002        (Resistances
2050 BV=5500                        (Blood volume
2060 RETURN
```

Figure 8.3 shows an example of inputting parameters where the default values are given under the heading LAST and the "?" is the point at which a value may be or may not be changed. All of the parameters were left unchanged except that the next simulation would be run with blood volume reduced from 5,500 to 5,000. Such might be the case for observing the steady-state mechanical consequences of a 500 ml hemorrhage.

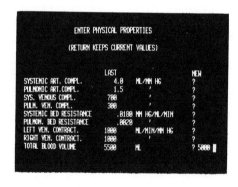

Figure 8.3. Photograph of a CRT display in which values of the physical parameters are being entered only if they differ from the present default values. The only item changed would be the blood volume which would be reduced to 5,000 ml. Note that absolute values and their units are given here.

An example of a routine to input changes from previously assigned values would consist, in part, of steps such as:

```
3000 REM     GET NEW PARAMETERS
3100 PRINT "LEFT VENTR CONTRACTILITY = ";K(1);:INPUT K(1)
3110 IF K(1) < 0 THEN PRINT "OUT OF RANGE": GOTO 3100
3300 ...
3400 REM                (Repeat for each parameter in turn
3900 ...
3999 RETURN
```

In this approach the student would have to have clear
instructions that the value of K(1) would be unchanged if the
RETURN key were to be pressed. With a little experience this
process gets to be a reflex so that it is possible to change
only one of the nine parameters very quickly and thus get to the
point of interest, the solution. Although for simplicity such
considerations are not included here, it is at this parameter
input stage where unrealistic results can be avoided either by
repeating the input statement or by giving error messages. In
the example of line 3110 above meaningless negative values of
contractility will be rejected. More elaborate tests could
ignore excessive values of some of the parameters and thus avoid
difficulties in final interpretations.

   Some versions of BASIC, such as Applesoft, require a
different tactic to retain default values since an input error
message is displayed if a RETURN is the response to an input
statement asking for the value of the variable. Without going
into the details here one method of achieving the desired
objective is to have the input statement ask for a string of
alphanumeric characters and then use the command for converting
this string into a numerical value. For example,

```
3100 INPUT A$
3120 IF VAL(A$) <>  0 THEN K(1)=VAL(A$)
```

Line 3100 asks for the value as a string labeled here by the
symbol A$. If the response to this query were a RETURN the
string would have a numerical value of zero and could be used to
indicate no change in the variable K(1). Values other than zero
would be used to modify that variable, as in line 3120. The use
of string variables as responses for input statements also
provides an opportunity to have the operator give a coded
command rather than a numerical value. For example, following
the above sequence with the line

```
3130 IF A$="RESTART" THEN GOTO 100
```

would allow the user to enter the command RESTART, exit from the
present operating sequence, and restart the simulation.

   A second comment regarding the input of system
parameters is that for this particular model all of the physical
properties except for blood volume are idealized abstractions
not encountered in practice. Although it is important for a
student to realize that the compliances of the venous
compartments are considerably greater than for the arterial
ones, the exact numerical values are not particulary meaningful.
Rather than ask the student to enter in exact numerical values
for each parameter it can be more expedient to have these
values, except for blood volume, normalized.

Thus one can explore the effects of 0.50 or 1.50 times normal peripheral resistance without being too concerned about their exact numerical values. Such a display is illustrated in Figure 8.I where the next simulation will be run with a peripheral resistance of 1.5 times the baseline value of 0.018. A routine to achieve this might consist of steps such as:

```
3000 REM    GET NEW PARAMETERS
3800 Z=R(1)/.018        (Z=temporary normalized default value
3310 INPUT  Z           (New or default normalized value
3820 R(1)=Z * .018      (New absolute value
3830 ...
3800 ...
3999 RETURN
```

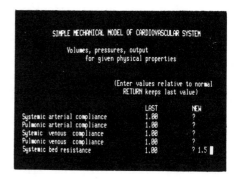

Figure 8.4. Inputting the parameters as normalized values rather than unfamiliar absolute values. For this simulation the systemic resistance will be 1.5 times the normal value.

In this method the normal value for each of the parameters would be part of the input subroutine, as the 0.018 in line 3800 above is used to compute a normalized default value for peripheral resistance. Line 3810 asks for a new resistance value in normalized form (1.0 being the reply for a normal value) or retains the default value. Then line 3820 changes this into an absolute value for computation purposes. One potential distraction which can be circumvented is that repeated operations such as these may produce coefficients as 0.999 or 1.001 through truncation errors.

THE SOLUTION

The essence of the simulation is contained in the portion involving the simultaneous solutions of the component relationships. In the listing of page 91 this subroutine is called at line 130. For the steady state the outputs of the two ventricles and the flows through the pulmonary and the systemic vascular beds are all equal to one another. This means that there are nine equations from Table 8.3 which are to be solved for the nine unknowns in Table 8.2.

There are a number of alternative methods for solving
this large number of simultaneous linear equations. Large
computer program libraries generally have maxtrix algebra
routines which could provide solutions by matrix inversion
techniques, but, this facility is not typical of microcomputer
versions of BASIC. Another approach would be to solve the
relations iteratively, starting with arbitrary initial values of
the variables and repeating the process until these no longer
change. This method is simple to program and to explain but
could be time consuming if the variables converge slowly toward
their final values.

The alternative chosen by the author is a
straight-forward Gaussian elimination method requiring
considerable algebra before programming is begun. In this
method eight of the variables are eliminated by combining the
nine equations until there is only one equation in one unknown,
the pulmonary venous volume VV(2) in terms of the physical
parameters. This value can be used to work back through the
reduced equations until all nine computed variables are found.
The correctness of the algebra always can be verified by seeing
that a set of computed values do indeed satisfy the individual
equations. The initial implementation of this method is tedious
and uninformative to document but once the program is written it
provides rapid solutions for that particular set of equations.

Table 8.4 gives the subroutine which calculates the
model's variables from the given physical parameters. For
manipulative and programming convenience the physical parameters
are combined into nine intermediate combinations denoted by
variables X1 through X9 in lines 1010 through 1090 of the
subroutine. These have no physiological meaning in themselves
but are merely intermediate coefficients involved in combining
the nine original equations. Similarly the four variables Y1
through Y4, defined in lines 1110 through 1140, are further
combinations which make it convenient to solve for the variable
VV(2) the pulmonary venous volume in line 1160. This value is
used to find systemic venous volume VV(1) in line 1170 and these
in turn are used to find the remaining variables in the
remaining lines of the subroutine.

It must be emphasized that the intermediate variables in
this subroutine apply only to the particular nine relationships
given in Table 8.4; any slight modification of any one of these
will require a whole new derivation. Upon exiting from the
given subroutine the values of cardiac output, vascular
pressures, and distribution of blood volume will be identified
for the particular contractilities, compliances, resistance, and
blood volume used in the calculations.

Table 8.4

BASIC subroutine for finding the steady-state solutions for the nine relationships given in Table 8.3 for the physical parameters defined in Table 8.1.

```
1000 REM  CALCULATE STEADY-STATE VALUES OF VARIABLES
1010 X1=(AC(1)*K(1)*R(1))/(VC(2)*(.01*R(1)*K(1)+1))
1020 X2=(AC(1))/(VC(1)*(.01*R(1)*K(1)+1))
1030 X3=(.01*100*K(1)*R(1)*AC(1))/(.01*R(1)*K(1)+1)
1040 X4=(AC(2)*K(2)*R(2))/(VC(1)*(.01*R(2)*K(2)+1))
1050 X5=(AC(2))/(VC(2)*(.01*K(2)*R(2)+1))
1060 X6=(.01*15*K(2)*R(2)*AC(2))/(.01*R(2)*K(2)+1)
1070 X7=(VC(1))/AC(1)
1080 X8=(VC(1)*R(1))/(AC(2)*R(2))
1090 X9=(VC(1)*R(1))/(VC(2)*R(2))
1100 :
1110 Y1=(X5*X8-X9+X7+X5*X7)/(1+X4*X8+X7+X4*X7)
1120 Y2=(BV*X7-X6*X7-X6*X8)/(1+X4*X8+X7+X4*X7)
1130 Y3=(X1+1+X5)/(X2+1+X4)
1140 Y4=(BV-X6-X3)/(X2+1+X4)
1150 :
1160 VV(2)=(Y2-Y4)/(Y1-Y3)       (Pulm ven vol
1170 VV(1)=Y2-VV(2)*Y1           (Syst ven vol
1180 AV(1)=X3+VV(1)*X2+VV(2)*X1  (Syst art vol
1190 AV(2)=BV-AV(1)-VV(1)-VV(2)  (Pulm art vol
1200 AP(1)=AV(1)/AC(1)           (Syst art press
1210 AP(2)=AV(2)/AC(2)           (Pulm art press
1220 VP(1)=VV(1)/VC(1)           (Syst ven press
1230 VP(2)=VV(2)/VC(2)           (Pulm ven press
1240 CO(1)=(AP(1)-VP(1))/R(1)    (Cardiac ouput
1250 RETURN
```

OUTPUT DISPLAYS

The form of the output displays will vary depending upon the version of BASIC and the CRT alphanumeric capabilities. One of the simpliest approaches is to have successive PRINT statments identify the variable and give its value with units one line at a time on either the CRT or a printer, such as

```
4000 REM   DISPLAY COMPUTED VALUES
4100 PRINT "CARDIAC OUTPUT = ";CO(1);" ML/MIN"
4200 PRINT "SYS. ART. PRESS.= ";AP(1); " MM HG"
4300 ...
4999 RETURN
```

One of the advantages of simulation on microcomputers is that their CRT´s can display output rapidly enough to hold the operator´s attention.    But with the typical 16 or 24 lines of characters it is necessary to organize the computed responses into a table format in order to make full use of the space available.  Illustrations will be given here for both kinds of computers.    Figure 8.3 is a photograph of an output of the static cardiovascular simulation on a CRT capable of displaying 16 lines of 64 characters.       After lines giving operating instructions, the student is presented the parameters by name one at a time along with the default value which will be retained if a RETURN key is pressed.    Typically the exercise requires only one or two of these parameters to be modfied and the new value is displayed along the right-hand edge of the table.    After the final parameter, blood volume, is entered the program makes the computations of steady-state variables according to the subroutine starting in line 3000.

In the example of Figure 8.5 the computed variables are displayed in three lines along the bottom of the screen while the top part retains both the previous and the newest values of the physical parameters.    The first line of computed values gives the systemic and pulmonic vascular volumes and pressures which would be expected normally.  These are the same for all simulations and serve as a basis of comparison.  The second line gives the values of these variables for the previous simulation using the parameters displayed in the upper middle column on the screen.  The bottom line gives the new simulation based upon the present values of the physical properties.  At this point it is possible to go on to another run with these same properties as default values (branch to line 120) or restart with normal values (branch to line 110) by pressing specific keys.

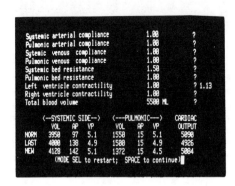

Figure 8.5. The results of two simulations as compared to the normally expected values in the model. This mimics essential hypertension by a combination of increased peripheral resistance and an increase in contractily as the result of ventricular hypertrophy.

In Figure 8.5 the first simulation changed only the systemic vascular resistance, increasing it by 50% over normal. The solution for this set of circumstances is those pressures and volumes and cardiac output in the line labeled "LAST".  Note

the rise in systemic arterial pressure and the fall in cardiac
output. In the second simulation the contractility was
increased by a value of 13% over normal. The line of computed
variables labeled "NEW" shows that with this simulation of
myocardial hypertrophy the cardiac output has been returned to
normal resting value but with further hypertension.

Figure 8.6 is a photograph of a similar output format
except that the absolute values of cardiovascular constants are
given. In the first simulation the left ventricular
contractility has been reduced and the major point to observe is
the shift of total blood volume into the pulmonary venous
compartment where it compromises pulmonary function. The
consequent increase in pressure filling the left ventricle
increases the end-diastolic volume and the heart is able to
moderate the fall in its output. The second simulation mimics
another feature of congestive failure by increasing the blood
volume. Note the further increase of pulmonary blood volume and
the return of cardiac output to a normal value. The display
permits the student to see the values of parameters for the two
situations and to compare their cardiovascular consequences with
the normal.

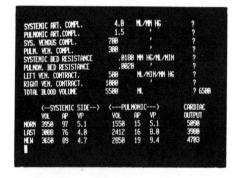

Figure 8.6. The results of
two simulations, the first
with decreased left
ventricular contractility, the
second with additional blood
volume. Note the large blood
volume in the pulmonary
vascular bed, mimicing the
conditions of congestive
failure.

For computer displays having 24 lines of 40 characters
each the information can be arranged on the CRT with alternative
formats. Figure 8.7 shows an arrangement which uses the Apple
II's abilily to place a text window in any area on the screen
without disturbing the surrounding text. This simulation uses
the same physical parameters as were used in the exercise of
Figure 8.5 in which systemic vascular resistance is at 1.5 times
normal on one iteration. The computed variables displayed apply
to that condition of the cardiovascular system. In the middle
of the screen a display window has been defined which is 7
characters wide and 14 lines tall into which desired changes of
the individual parameters may be entered. After the final one,
blood volume, is entered the default parameters and computed
variables are updated and the display is then ready for the next

set of entries.  The Applesoft BASIC listing for this program is
given in the Chapter Appendix.

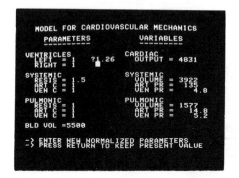

Fig.  8.7.  A display format
for a CRT with 24 lines of 40
characters.  The  computed
variables  correspond  to  the
normalized  parameters given.
The  operator  is  answering
queries  for  the  next
iteration.  The text stays in
place on the screen while the
numerical  values  are  placed
in  program-controlled window
areas.

        In these tabular displays it is necessary to take special
steps to have the computed variables line  up  neatly  within  a
limited    space.    Some  versions  of  BASIC  contain  special
formatting statements which  permit  this.    For  example,  the
statement

        4100  PRINT USING "###."; AP(1):

will  round  off  the  fractional parts of the computed arterial
pressure.  The same result can be achieved with  greater  effort
in    BASIC's    without    this    feature  by  special  formatting
subroutines based on either of two  approaches.    The  computed
variable can be converted to a string variable any part of which
may be printed a  character  at  a  time.    Alternatively,  the
integer    function  can  be  combined  with  multiplication  and
division of powers of ten to retain only the desired digits.

        Microcomputers  with  graphic  capabilities  can  provide
displays  of  the  model's  functional  relationships  so    that
students  can  visualize  modifications  in cardiac and vascular
functions as their parameters are changed.  For  nine  equations
with  nine  variables  this  would  involve 9-dimensional space.
Textbooks  of  physiology  generally  emphasize  two  of    these
variables   with graphs,   the  important relationship between the
low-pressure filling the ventricles and the   ventricular   output
and   the   fact   that   this output in turn determines the filling
pressure.   Intersections of these functions define the operating
points  of  the  total  system  for  a  given  set  of  physical
properties.

        Figure  8.8   illustrates   such   a  graph displayed on an
Apple II.  It is important to  keep  in  mind   that the functional

relationships shown here are approximations in two ways. First, they are based on assumptions for linearity for computational simplicity. Secondly, these functions also do not allow for the fact that the arterial pressures are another changing variable which will also change the ventricular function curves. But, since the afterload effects are relatively small, the graphs are useful within the limits of their resolution.

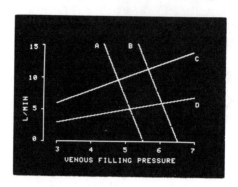

Fig. 8.8. Graphic displays of ventricular function curves, lines C and D, and of venous return curves, lines A and B. The points where these lines intercept define the cardiac output and venous pressure for given physical conditions. Lines A and D are for normal, B is for elevated blood volume, and C is for increased contractility.

The relationships given by lines C and D in Figure 8.8 correspond to the ventricular function curves with venous filling pressure as the independent variable and cardiac output as the dependent variable. These lines, sometimes referred to as "Starling curves", are not linear in practice but reach a plateau and even descend at large extenstion pressures. In this figure the contractility for function C was increased from that for normal approximated by function D.

In the steady state, in which cardiac output and venous return are equal, as the flow rates are increased blood volume is moved from the venous to the arterial segments commenserate with the pressure gradient between them. Though the venous pressure changes are slight they are very significant in determining the end-diastolic ventricular volume. Lines A and B in Figure 8.8 are representations of these vascular functions, often called "venous return curves." At zero cardiac output their x-intercepts indicate the mean circulatory pressures as determined primarily by total blood volume and vascular compliances. The function at line B was obtained for elevated blood volume.

As noted above the intercepts of pairs of lines
establish approximations to the values of the system variables
as computed by solving the nine equations with the corresponding
physical parameters. For example, the intercept of lines A and
D establishes the normal cardiac output and venous filling
pressure. With increased contractility, as plotted by line A,
the intercept corresponds to higher cardiac output at lower
venous pressure. The intercept of lines C and B illustrates the
mechanical conditions following infusion of blood and increased
ventricular contractility.

## STEADY-STATE EXERCISES

The purpose of this section is to use the described
mechanical model of the cardiovascular system in the context of
teaching exercises. A major objective is to illustrate that
system variables such as cardiac output and arterial pressure
are determined by the mechanical properties of both the heart
and the vascular beds. The negative feedback or homeostatic
property introduced by the Starling Law gives an intrinsic
mechanical stability, equating the average outputs of the two
hearts without requiring neural regulation. The model
illustrates that the effects of changing one parameter are
moderated by the interactive mechanical coupling between heart
and vessels. Furthermore, certain variables are more easily
influenced by changes in specific physical properties than by
changes in the others.

The sequence which follows is that which the author
uses. This begins by looking at the distribution of blood
volume with the ventricles stopped and then observing that with
increasing contractility there is a shift of blood volume from
the venous to the arterial side, lowering the venous and raising
the arterial pressures around a baseline level called the "mean
circulatory pressure". The intent is to use this as a guide for
an instructor to develop a specific teaching protocol according
to his/her particular approach and facilities.

## VARIATIONS IN CONTRACTILITY

In this model contractility encompasses both the
property of myocardial strength (the usual connotation) and the
heart rate. The former can be influenced by the cardiac mass,
excitation efficiency, metabolism, and valvular function while
both aspects can be influenced by autonomic and endocrine
control.

By setting the contractilities to zero one can observe
the  static conditions simulated with no gravitational gradients
of a subject in the supine position. Pressures will  be  uniform
in  all  vascular  compartments at the mean circulatory pressure
(about 5.5 mm Hg in this model) and the total blood volume  will
be  distributed  according  to the compliances of the individual
compartments.  It should be noted that a significant portion  of
the total volume is in the systemic venous segment.  The factors
which influence  the  base-line  pressure  can  be  explored  by
manipulating  blood volume and venous compliances one at a time.
Also  note  that  vascular  resistances  and  ventricular
contractilities are not involved since there is no flow then.

The next step is to  increase  both  contractilities  in
steps  of  0.25  times  normal  and  observe  the large rises in
arterial pressures and slight falls in venous pressures.   With
increasing  cardiac function there is a shift of volume from the
venous side into the arterial side with  the  pressure  changes
being  correlated  with  the  differences  in compliances of the
associated  vessels.   The  magnitude  of  the  arterial-venous
gradients  are  those  which provide vascular bed flows to match
the cardiac outputs. The  degree  of  these  gradients  can  be
correlated  with  the  magnitude  of  the  associated  vascular
resistances.

Either  right or left heart failures can be simulated by
changing the appropriate contractility. The display of  Figure
8.6  illustrates  the condition when left heart contractility is
set to 0.5 with normal total blood volume.   There is a shift of
over  800  ml  from  the systemic to the pulmonic side. This is
chacteristic of congestive failure and its  associated  dyspnea.
Besides  this  clinical  aspect the following regulatory feature
should be examined.  Though the contractility is reduced to  50%
the  cardiac  output is about 80% of normal.  This is because as
output is reduced the increase  in  steady-state  venous  volume
causes  the  venous  filling  pressure  to  be elevated from the
normal 5.1, providing  a compensating factor aiding  ventricular
filling,  and  thus output.  This is an example of the fact that
negative feedback reduces the overall effects of changes in  the
parameters  of the components in the control loop.  If the right
ventriclar function is reduced and that of the  left  is  normal
there  is  a shift in volume to the systemic side but because of
the large venous compliance the  pressure  rise  there  is  less
significant and the cardiac compensation is less pronounced.

To pursue the congestive failure example a step further,
the  bottom  line in Figure 8.6 applies to a simulation in which
fluid retention is simulated by increasing the blood  volume  to
6500  ml.   A  significant  part  of  this  volume  ends in the
pulmonary bed, further compromising pulmonary function, but with
further  cardiac  compensation because of better filling of the
left ventricle.  In life this pulmonary vascular volume increase

may raise pulmonary pressures sufficiently to produce  pulmonary
edema   Also, the myocardium may be overextended so that further
increases  in  end-diastolic  volumes  actually  decrease   left
ventricle output.


CHANGES IN VASCULAR RESISTANCES

        This model lumps all of the peripheral vascular pathways
into a single equivalent resistance so that the specific effects
of  changing  the resistances of single organ systems can not be
done directly.  Nevertheless  it  is  possible  to  examine  the
consequences  of  the well-known increase in total resistance in
essential hypertension and the decrease with  exercise,  anemia,
and  arterial-venous  anastomoses.   The pulmonary vascular bed
resistance is often considered to be determined primarily by the
passive  mechanical  recruitment  and  distension  of  vascular
pathways with small increases in pulmonary  arterial  pressures.
Since this model considers the resistance to be constant it will
be necessary for the operator to make allowances  for  decreased
resistance at higher pulmonary pressures.

        Upon decreasing both the systemic and pulmonary vascular
resistances  to  some  value such as 0.5 times normal it will be
noted that there are only slight changes  in  the  blood  volume
distribution  and  venous  pressures but that there is a fall in
the arterial pressures. Because of  the  mechanical  homeostasis
the  cardiac  output does not double but increases by only a few
percent.  Systemic arterial  pressure,  on  the  other  hand  is
reduced  significantly.   This  illustrates  the  fact that the
mechanical consequences of changes in vascular resistance,  both
increases  and  decreases,  have  their greatest effect upon the
arterial pressures and less upon the ventricular outputs.  It is
true that the arterial pressure afterload influence upon cardiac
output is determined by the sensitivity coefficient  used  (0.01
in  this  model)  but  it  is  also  true  that  this effect is
relatively small compared to the venous pressure effects.

        The  clinical  conditions  of pulmonary hypertension and
essential hypertension can be  simulated  by  increases  in  the
resistance of the appropriate vascular bed.  In both cases there
is a rise in arterial pressure and  a  slight  fall  in  cardiac
output  which  can  be brought back to  normal by increasing the
ventricular contractility to mimic hypertrophy of that  chamber.
This  simulation  is  displayed  in  Figure  8.5 where increased
systemic resistance  and  left  ventricular  contractility  give
normal  cardiac  output  but elevated arterial pressure.  Though
the model is not this refined it should not be  overlooked  that
even  with  normal cardiac output being restored it will be at a
large metabolic cost because of the high afterloading.   Indeed,
that  metabolic load upon the myocardium may have stimulated the
hypertrophy.

An interesting sidelight is to exchange the systemic and pulmonary resistances by entering values of 0.1 for the former and 10.0 for the latter. For this condition the cardiac output is about normal but the systemic and pulmonic arterial pressures are exchanged. Of course exchanging the systemic arterial and venous compliances will not exchange the pressures in these vessels because there must always be a forward gradient, but such a manuever does show that arterial pressure is drastically reduced with large values of compliance.


COMPLIANCE CHANGES


In actual fact vessel compliances vary markedly with vessel pressures and with sympathetic activity. Since this models utilizes constant compliances it can predict only the general direction of changes expected for the cardiovascular pressures and flows. Decreasing the systemic arterial compliance to 0.5 normal has a minor influence upon mean arterial pressure itself (the influence upon the systolic pressure would be another matter) but the shift of some blood to the venous side can account for some of the increase in cardiac output. This effect is minor because of the relatively small volume of the arterial segment. On the other hand reducing the system venous compliance to 0.5 normal shifts a significant amount of blood into the other compartments and increases venous filling pressures, cardiac outputs and arterial pressures. This would illustrate the effects of sympathetic "tightening up" of the systemic venous reservoir, including the spleen.


BLOOD VOLUME CHANGES


Increases and decreases of blood volume, as from infusion or hemorrhage respectively, are reflected mechanically by changes in the mean circulatory pressure, vascular pressures, and cardiac outputs. For this model with constant compliances there is no shifting of the fractional distribution of blood volume between compartments. We shall see a more informative role for volume changes in the transient model to be described later in this chapter.


EXERCISE


The conditions for exercise can be approximated by increases in ventricular contractilities and decreases in vascular resistances. For example, both contractilities can be increased to five times normal to reflect a change in both heart rate and actual myocardial strength. Systemic resistance can be decreased to 0.25 to reflect the overwhelming metabolic vasodilation characteristic of skeletal muscle activity. The pulmonary resistance can be set to 0.25 because of the passive effects of a slightly elevated pulmonary arterial pressure. When these particular illustrative values are used it will be observed that blood volume distribution and venous pressures are about the same, that there is a slight rise in arterial pressures and that cardiac output increases to almost five times the value for normal conditions.

```
┌─────────────────────────┐
│  TRANSIENT SOLUTIONS     │
└─────────────────────────┘
```

        Insight about how the cardiovascular system achieves its mechanical stability, with the outputs of the two ventricles being equal on the average, can be gained by following the transient solution to a small, sudden change of one of the parameters or of one of the variables. The illustration given here involes setting some initial set of physical parameters, using these to solve for the steady-state distribution of blood volume as before, and then observing the temporal changes in the computed variables following the infusion or hemorrhage of a small amount of the systemic venous blood volume. This produces a temporary difference in outputs from the two ventricles which gradually converge upon the new steady-state conditions appropriate for the change in total blood volume. This convergence to a new steady state following a disturbance of any of the parameters or computed variables is evidence of the stability introduced by the negative feedback of this homestatic system. The exercise also illustrates the most elementary method of simulating the transient solutions of a dynamic process described by a differential equation -- a mechanical analog for visualizing applied mathematics.

        The computational step that has to be introduced consists of setting up and solving differential equations containing the manipulated variable. Our presentation involves simple Euler, or rectangular, integration of the vascular compartmental volumes updated at time increments small enough that the flows into and out of these segments can be approximated as constant. At periodic intervals the two ventricular outputs, along with vascular volumes and pressures are displayed on the CRT in tabular form so that a student can follow the manner of the redistribution of total blood volume among the compartments. As was mentioned previously these mechanical transients are first-order exponentials and graphic displays do not reveal the numerical details of the process as well as does the tabular presentation which is given. In more elaborate simulations involving nonlinear pressure-volume curves and parameter modifications the graphic solutions could provide considerable information.

Before getting into the details of the present program it is advantageous to see the display of its results. In operation the student first sets the initial cardiovascular properties, as was done in Figure 8.4. Then, as in Figure 8.9A, the steady-state vascular volumes are displayed and the desired disturbance of the systemic venous volume is entered, such as the indicated loss of 500 ml of blood. The simulation of the first ten seconds of the transient response is given in Figure 8.9B.

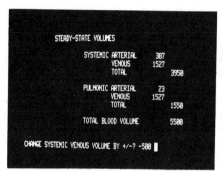
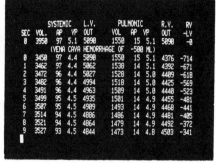

Fig. 8.9.  A) The steady-state distribution of blood volume for the properties selected in Figure 8.4. The disturbance is the loss of 500 ml from the systemic venous compartment. B) The volumes, vascular pressures, and ventricle outputs before and after the disturbance. The reduction in pressure filling the right ventricle reduces the output of the right heart but that from the left ventricle remains the same. In successive seconds this difference in outputs from the two ventricles shifts progressively less blood from the pulmonic to the systemic side until a new steady state is reached.


In the display of Figure 8.9B the pressures and volumes of the systemic and pulmonic beds are given along with the outputs of the two ventricles and the difference between these two outputs. The first line shows these values for the initial steady state. Subsequent lines follow the new values for successive seconds. The computations of new vascular volumes and pressures actually are done for 0.1 second increments with every 10th one displayed for reading convenience. We shall now describe the computer programs which accomplish this simulation and then return to discuss the physiological significance of the columns of numbers.

THE SOLUTION

    Table 8.4 gives the main routine for initializing and
updating the vascular volumes and pressures. This calls several
subroutines which perform more specialized functions and which
are described separately in more detail, except for those
relatinJ tI output formats which vary with the version of BASIC
and computer being used. Lines 220 through 280 establish the
initial parameters and value of the disturbance. Line 300 sets
the variable T for time equal to zero. Line 310 sets the
computation increment DT equal to 1/600 minutes (0.1 sec) since
the units of flow are in ml/min. Once these initial conditions
are set the actual simulation runs in lines 330-390 in which new
volumes, pressures, and flow rates are computed for each 0.1 sec
and displayed for each second.

---

Table 8.4

Main routine for transient solutions of the simple
mechanical model of the cardiovascular system. This
generates a tabular listing of vascular volumes, and
pressures following a sudden change in systemic venous
blood volume. It illustrates the manner by which the
blood volume is redistributed until a new steady state
is established.


```
200 REM     TRANSIENTS FOLLOWING VENOUS VOLUME CHANGES
210 :
220 GOSUB 2000              (Set normal, default values
230 GOSUB 3000              (Establish initial parameters
240 GOSUB 1000              (Find steady-state variables
250 GOSUB 5000              (Display initial volumes
260 INPUT "CHANGE IN VENOUS VOLUME"; DV
270 VV(1) = VV(1) + DV
280 BV    = BV    + DV
290 :
300 T  = 0                  (Initial variable time
310 DT = 1/600              (Comp.increment = 0.1 sec.
320 :
330 FOR TT= 1 TO 10         (Counts computations/display
340    GOSUB 6000           (Calculate pressures, flows
350    GOSUB 7000           (Update volumes from flows
360    NEXT TT              (Increment counter
380 GOSUB 8000             (Print every 10 iterations
390 GOSUB 330              (Repeat for next 10
```

The setting up of the initial parameters and steady-state values in subroutines at lines 2000, 3000, and 1000 is identical as given before. The subroutine at line 5000, not given here, is an option which tells the student just how the blood volume is distributed initially. The input statement in line 260 requests the disturbance of the systemic venous volume desired, denoted as DV here. The bottom line of Figure 8.9A displays this stage of the process. In line 270 the new value of this variable, VV(1), is set by adding DV to the steady-state value. In line 280 the new blood volume BV is similarly established.

The variable TT is used to count the number of computations between each displayed line. Every 10th iteration the program goes to the printing subroutine in line 8000. For those computers where the CRT lines continually scroll up it is necessary to periodically repeat the column headings by including an additional counter and command statements. In the Apple II it is possible to fix the column heading at the top of the screen and have successive lines of computation scroll under these labels. Because of this variance among computers the details are not pursued here.

The subroutine starting at line 6000 and called from within the iteration loop at line 340 uses the existing vascular volumes to calculate the pressures in each vascular compartment. These in turn are used to calculate the cardiac outputs from the respective ventricles and the flows through the pulmonic and systemic vascular circuits according to the relationships defined in Table 8.3.

```
6000 REM    PRESSURES AND FLOWS FOR PRESENT VOLUMES
6010 AP(1) = AV(1)/AC(1):  AP(2) = AV(2)/AC(2)
6020 VP(1) = VV(1)/VC(1):  VP(2) = VV(2)/VC(2)
6030 CO(1) = K(1)*VP(2)  - 0.01*K(1)*(AP(1)-100)
6040 CO(2) = K(2)*VP(1)  - 0.01*K(2)*(AP(2)-15)
6050 FL(1) = (AP(1)-VP(1))/R(1)
6060 FL(2) = (AP(2)-VP(2))/R(2)
6070 RETURN
```

Once the pressures and flows have been established for the existing volumes it is possible to calculate new volumes of each vascular compartment by adding the amount of blood which enters during a finite time and subtracting the amount which leaves during the interval. If the computation increment taken is sufficiently short these influxes and effluxes can be considered as constants determined by the present cardiac outputs and vascular bed flows just calculated. The value of DT = 0.1 second seems to be a reasonable compromise between accuracy and speed for the teaching objectives, but more sophisticated numerical integration methods are, of course, available. For the rectangular integration method used here the change in systemic arterial volume DA(1) is found by the net result of

$$DA(1) = CO(1)*DT - FL(1)*DT$$
    net        flow in       flow out

and the change in systemic venous volume DV(1) is found by the net result of

$$DV(1) = FL(1)*DT - CO(2)*DT$$
    net        flow in   - flow out

The subroutine using these integrations is

```
7000 REM    UPDATE VOLUMES FROM FLOWS DURING DT
7010 AV(1) = AV(1) + CO(1)*DT - FL(1)*DT
7020 VV(1) = VV(1) + FL(1)*DT - CO(2)*DT
7030 AV(2) = AV(2) + CO(2)*DT - FL(2)*DT
7040 VV(2) = BV - AV(1) - AV(2) - VV(1)
7050 T = T + DT
7060 RETURN
```

In this subroutine line 7010 finds the new systemic arterial volume by adding the amount which enters from the left ventricle during increment DT and subtracting the amount which leaves through the systemic vascular bed. Lines 7020 and 7030 similary update the systemic venous and the pulmonic arterial vascular volumes. In line 7040 the pulmonic venous volume is calculated by subtracting the other three volumes from the total blood volume in order to assure conservation of the total amount of blood during repeated imprecise computations. In line 7060 the cummulative time is updated by the computation increment.

Elementary as it may sound here, these steps are the essence of the dynamic aspects of physiology and the solutions of differential equations. Most of the body's variables are in some dynamic equilibra determined by a balance of factors adding to them and factors diminishing them. The imbalance between these factors forces the variable to change. Differential equations are simply explicit statements of those factors adding and those removing, stated in terms of known parameters and of other variables in the system. Computer similation provides a convenient means of doing this bookkeeping and offers advantages over formal integrative methods in that thresholds and nonlinearities are handled by including conditional command statements and products of variables.

The subroutine which prints each line of the simulation
depends upon the length of a CRT line of characters and upon the
method of formatting variables in BASIC. For the CP/M Microsoft
BASIC and the 64-character display used in Figure 8.9B the
subroutine consists of

```
8000 REM      PRINT LINE OF VALUES ON CRT
8010 A$=
"##    ####  ### ##.#  ####      ####  ### ##.# #### #####"
8020 PRINT USING A$;T*60;AV(1)+VV(1);AP(1);VP(1);CO(1);
        AV(2)+VV(2)+AP(2);VP(2);CO(2);CO(2)-CO(1)
8030 RETURN
```

Line 8010 sets up the string variable A$ to lay out the format
of the successive variables and the spacing between them on a
64-character line. Line 8020 prints these variables according
to that format. Computers with 24 lines of 40 characters, such
as the Apple II, must limit the number of variables or their
precision as displayed on each line.


EXAMINING THE TRANSIENT

Let us now look at the mechanical processes involved
which operated as soon as the 500 ml of blood was removed from
the systemic vascular compartment in the previous illustration.
The reader should refer to Figure 8.9B during this discussion.
This is a mathematical hemorrhage in that any real one would
occur over some finite time. With the sudden drop in venous
volume from 3,563 to 3,063 ml there is a correspondingly rapid
fall in systemic venous pressure from 5.1 to 4.4 mm Hg. Since
our model does not include systolic and diastolic ventricular
events the simplification merely says that there is a rapid fall
in right ventricular output from 5,090 ml/min to 4,376 ml/min.
Meanwhile the factors influencing left ventricle output have not
yet had time to change so that this side of the heart continues
with the initial rate of 5,090 ml/min. This imbalance of
outputs between the two sides of the heart provides the driving
force to shift blood from the pulmonary circuit into the
systemic side and to restore a balance of fluxes into and out of
each of the vascular compartments.

Over some finite time during this transient there will
be a reduced flow into the pulmonary artery from the right
ventricle but the exiting flow through the pulmonary resistance
will remain about the same. This will cause the pulmonary
arterial pressure to gradually fall as is seen in the tabular
presentation. Similarly with less blood leaving the systemic
venous compartment but about the same flow into it from the
systemic capillaries there is a gradual increase in systemic
venous volume and pressure as can be followed in Figure 8.9B.

As these volumes gradually readjust the extent of the driving forces are reduced in an exponential manner with a time constant dominated by the mechanical compliances and resistances. As was stated previously this readjustment is slow in the model because no allowance is made for neurally-evoked changes such as increases in contractility and reduced venous compliance. Figure 8.10 shows the simulation for 40-50 seconds by which time the shift in blood into the systemic venous system is evident from the increase in its pressure and the corresponding decreases in pressures in the other compartment. The original loss of 500 ml now is being shared by all vascular compartments. Eventually a new steady-state is reached in which outputs of the right and left ventricles are equal to each other, but less than before there was a blood loss.

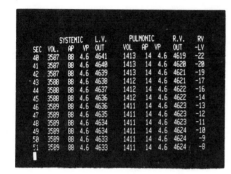

| SEC | SYSTEMIC VOL. | AP | VP | L.V. OUT | PULMONIC VOL | AP | VP | R.V. OUT | RV -LV |
|---|---|---|---|---|---|---|---|---|---|
| 40 | 3587 | 88 | 4.6 | 4641 | 1413 | 14 | 4.6 | 4619 | -22 |
| 41 | 3587 | 88 | 4.6 | 4640 | 1413 | 14 | 4.6 | 4620 | -20 |
| 42 | 3587 | 88 | 4.6 | 4639 | 1413 | 14 | 4.6 | 4621 | -19 |
| 43 | 3588 | 88 | 4.6 | 4638 | 1412 | 14 | 4.6 | 4621 | -17 |
| 44 | 3588 | 88 | 4.6 | 4637 | 1412 | 14 | 4.6 | 4622 | -16 |
| 45 | 3588 | 88 | 4.6 | 4636 | 1412 | 14 | 4.6 | 4622 | -14 |
| 46 | 3589 | 88 | 4.6 | 4636 | 1411 | 14 | 4.6 | 4623 | -13 |
| 47 | 3589 | 88 | 4.6 | 4635 | 1411 | 14 | 4.6 | 4623 | -12 |
| 48 | 3589 | 88 | 4.6 | 4634 | 1411 | 14 | 4.6 | 4623 | -11 |
| 49 | 3589 | 88 | 4.6 | 4634 | 1411 | 14 | 4.6 | 4624 | -10 |
| 50 | 3589 | 88 | 4.6 | 4633 | 1411 | 14 | 4.6 | 4624 | -9 |
| 51 | 3589 | 88 | 4.6 | 4633 | 1411 | 14 | 4.6 | 4624 | -8 |

Fig. 8.10. A continuation of the simulation started in Figure 8.9B. There has been a shift of blood into the systemic circuit that has partially restored venous pressure there but at the expense of volumes and pressures in the other compartments. Note that right and left outputs are becoming more nearly equal.

The transient response could be made much more informative by having the model include more realistic factors such as heart rate changes and pulsatile pressures. It has been said that a mathematical model is useful if it stimulates someone to produce a more comprehensive one. Perhaps the simplicity of this model presented in this chapter may be useful to some readers just becoming interested in microcomputer simulation. Hopefully, there will also be an audience of knowledgeable cardiovascular physiologists who will be sufficiently offended by this model's crudeness that they will develop better ones for distribution to the growing group of microcomputer users.

REFERENCES

Beeuwkes. R., and N. Braslow:   The  cardiovascular  trainer:   A
real  time  physiological  simulator.   Physiology Teacher 3:4-7
(1971).

Coleman, T. G., R. d. Manning, Jr., R. A. Norman, Jr., and A. C.
Guyton:  Control  of  cardiac  output  by  regional  blood  flow
distribututiion.  Annals of Biomed. Engr. 2:149-163 (1974).

Defares, J. G., J. J. Osborn  and  H.  H.  Hara:    Theoretical
synthesis  of  the  cardiovascular  system.    Study I:    the
controlled system.  Acta Pharmacol Neerl. 12:189-265 (1963).

Dickinson, C. J., C. E. Goldsmith, and D. L. Sackett:  MACMAN: A
digital computer model for teaching  some  basic  principles  of
hemodynamics. J. Clin. Comp. 2:42-50 (1973).

Grodins, F. S.:    Integrative  cardiovascular  physiology:   a
mathematical synthesis of cardiac and blood vessel hemodynamics.
Quart. Rev. Biol. 34:93-116 (1959).

Guyton,  A.  C.:    Determination  of cardiac output by equating
venous return curves with cardiac  response  curves.    Physiol.
Rev. 35:123-129 (1955).

Guyton, A. C., T. G. Coleman, and H. J. Granger:   Circulation:
overall regulation.  Ann. Rev. Physiol. 34:13-46 (1972).

Katz, S., R. G. Hollingsworth, J. G. Blackburn, and H. T.
Carter:  Computer  simulation  in  the  physiology  student
laboratory.  Physiol. Teacher, Physiologist 21:41-44 (1978).

CHAPTER APPENDIX

The program listing on  the  next  three  pages  is the
Applesoft  BASIC  version used in generating the static solution
display as given in Figure 8.7.  The sequence  is  the  same  as
that  used  in  the  illustrative routines in this chapter.  The
subroutines in lines 2500, 2800, and 3000 make use of the  Apple
II  variable  text  window,  the  limits of which are POKED into
memory starting at address 32.  Thus the program  illustrates  a
format  for  replacing variables while the column and row titles
stay fixed on the CRT display.

```
100  REM   CARDIOVASCULAR MECHANICS MODEL FOR APPLE-II COMPUTER
101  REM    REQUESTS HEART AND VESSEL PHYSICAL PARAMETERS
102  REM    DISPLAYS STEADY-STATE PRESSURES, VOLUMES, OUTPUT
103  :
104  :
105  GOSUB 1500: REM --CRT TABLE TEXT
110  GOSUB 2000: REM --SET DEFAULT PARAMETERS
112  GOSUB 1000: REM --CALCULATE NORMAL VARIABLES
113  :
115  GOSUB 2500: REM --DISPLAY PARAMETERS  <------------
120  GOSUB 2800: REM --DISPLAY VARIABLES
125  GOSUB 3000: REM --GET NEW PARAMETERS
130  GOSUB 1000: REM --SOLVE FOR VARIABLES
135  GOTO 115: REM   --REPEAT FOR NEW PARAMETERS ------->
140  :
150  :
160  :
1000 : REM   CALCULATE 9 S-S VARIABLES FROM 9 EQUATIONS
1001 :
1010 X1 = (AC(1) * K(1) * R(1))
1015 X1 = X1 / (VC(2) * (.01 * R(1) * K(1) + 1))
1020 X2 = (AC(1)) / (VC(1) * (.01 * R(1) * K(1) + 1))
1030 X3 = (.01 * 100 * K(1) * R(1) * AC(1))
1035 X3 = X3 / (.01 * R(1) * K(1) + 1)
1040 X4 = (AC(2) * K(2) * R(2))
1045 X4 = X4 / (VC(1) * (.01 * R(2) * K(2) + 1))
1050 X5 = (AC(2)) / (VC(2) * (.01 * K(2) * R(2) + 1))
1060 X6 = (.01 * 15 * K(2) * R(2) * AC(2))
1065 X6 = X6 / (.01 * R(2) * K(2) + 1)
1070 X7 = (VC(1)) / AC(1)
1080 X8 = (VC(1) * R(1)) / (AC(2) * R(2))
1090 X9 = (VC(1) * R(1)) / (VC(2) * R(2))
1100 :
1110 Y1 = (X5 * X8 - X9 + X7 + X5 * X7)
1115 Y1 = Y1 / (1 + X4 * X8 + X7 + X4 * X7)
1120 Y2 = (BV * X7 - X6 * X7 - X6 * X8)
1125 Y2 = Y2 / (1 + X4 * X8 + X7 + X4 * X7)
1130 Y3 = (X1 + 1 + X5) / (X2 + 1 + X4)
1140 Y4 = (BV - X6 - X3) / (X2 + 1 + X4)
1150 :
1160 VV(2) = (Y2 - Y4) / (Y1 - Y3)
1170 VV(1) = Y2 - VV(2) * Y1
1180 AV(1) = X3 + VV(1) * X2 + VV(2) * X1
1190 AV(2) = BV - AV(1) - VV(1) - VV(2)
1200 AP(1) = AV(1) / AC(1)
1210 AP(2) = AV(2) / AC(2)
1220 VP(1) = VV(1) / VC(1)
1230 VP(2) = VV(2) / VC(2)
1240 CO(1) = (AP(1) - VP(1)) / R(1)
1250  RETURN
1260 :
1265 :
```

```
1500   REM     PUT TABLE TEXT ONTO CRT SCREEN
1510   :
1520   TEXT : HOME : HTAB 3
1530   PRINT "MODEL FOR CARDIOVASCULAR MECHANICS"
1540   PRINT
1550   HTAB 5: PRINT "PARAMETERS";
1560   HTAB 25: PRINT "VARIABLES"
1570   HTAB 5: PRINT "----------";
1575   HTAB 25: PRINT "---------"
1580   PRINT
1590   PRINT "VENTRICLES";
1600   HTAB 22: PRINT "CARDIAC"
1610   PRINT "  LEFT  =";
1620   HTAB 23: PRINT " OUTPUT ="
1630   PRINT "  RIGHT ="
1640   PRINT
1650   PRINT "SYSTEMIC";: HTAB 22
1660   PRINT "SYSTEMIC"
1670   PRINT "  RESIS =";
1680   HTAB 24: PRINT "VOLUME ="
1690   PRINT "  ART C =";: HTAB 24
1700   PRINT "ART PR ="
1710   PRINT "  VEN C =";: HTAB 24
1720   PRINT "VEN PR =": PRINT
1730   PRINT "PULMONIC";: HTAB 22
1740   PRINT "PULMONIC"
1750   PRINT "  RESIS =";: HTAB 24
1760   PRINT "VOLUME ="
1770   PRINT "  ART C =";: HTAB 24
1780   PRINT "ART PR ="
1790   PRINT "  VEN C =";: HTAB 24
1800   PRINT "VEN PR =": PRINT
1820   PRINT "BLD VOL ="
1830   PRINT : PRINT
1840   PRINT "-- ENTER NEW NORMALIZED PARAMETERS"
1860   PRINT "-- PRESS RETURN TO KEEP PRESENT VALUE";
1870   RETURN
1880   :
1890   :
1900   :
2000   REM     SET DEFAULT PARAMETERS
2005   :
2010   K(1) = 1000:K(2) = 1000
2020   AC(1) = 4:AC(2) = 1.5
2030   VC(1) = 700:VC(2) = 300
2040   R(1) = 0.018:R(2) = 0.002
2050   BV = 5500
2060   RETURN
2070   :
2080   :
```

```
2500   REM   DISPLAY NORMALIZED PARAMETERS IN CRT WINDOW
2501   :
2510   POKE 33,6: POKE 32,10: POKE 34,6: POKE 35,21: HOME
2530   PRINT  INT (100 * K(1) / 1000) / 100
2540   PRINT  INT (100 * K(2) / 1000) / 100
2550   PRINT : PRINT
2560   PRINT  INT (100 * R(1) / .018 + .5) / 100
2570   PRINT  INT (100 * AC(1) / 4) / 100
2590   PRINT  INT (100 * VC(1) / 700) / 100
2600   PRINT : PRINT
2610   PRINT  INT (100 * R(2) / .002) / 100
2620   PRINT  INT (100 * AC(2) / 1.5) / 100
2630   PRINT  INT (100 * VC(2) / 300) / 100
2650   POKE 32,9: PRINT : PRINT  INT (BV)
2660   RETURN
2670   :
2800   REM    DISPLAY VARIABLES IN CRT WINDOW
2801   :
2810   POKE 33,7: POKE 32,32: HOME
2820   VTAB 7: PRINT  INT (CO(1))
2830   VTAB 11: PRINT  INT (AV(1) + VV(1))
2840   PRINT " "; INT (AP(1))
2850   PRINT "   "; INT (10 * VP(1) + .5) / 10
2860   VTAB 16: PRINT  INT (AV(2) + VV(2))
2870   PRINT " "; INT (10 * AP(2) + .5) / 10
2880   PRINT "   "; INT (10 * VP(2) + .5) / 10
2890   RETURN
2900   :
3000   REM   ASK FOR NEW PARAMETERS; RETURN = DEFAULT
3005   :
3010   POKE 33,6: POKE 32,14: POKE 34,6: HOME
3020   INPUT A$
3030   IF  VAL (A$) <  > 0 THEN K(1) =  VAL (A$) * 1000
3040   INPUT A$
3050   IF  VAL (A$) <  > 0 THEN K(2) =  VAL (A$) * 1000
3060   VTAB 11: INPUT A$
3070   IF  VAL (A$) <  > 0 THEN R(1) =  VAL (A$) * .018
3080   INPUT A$
3090   IF  VAL (A$) <  > 0 THEN AC(1) =  VAL (A$) * 4
3100   INPUT A$
3110   IF  VAL (A$) <  > 0 THEN VC(1) =  VAL (A$) * 700
3120   VTAB 16: INPUT A$
3130   IF  VAL (A$) <  > 0 THEN R(2) =  VAL (A$) * .002
3140   INPUT A$
3150   IF  VAL (A$) <  > 0 THEN AC(2) =  VAL (A$) * 1.5
3160   INPUT A$
3170   IF  VAL (A$) <  > 0 THEN VC(2) =  VAL (A$) * 300
3180   VTAB 20: INPUT A$
3200   IF  VAL (A$) <  > 0 THEN BV =  VAL (A$)
3210   RETURN
```

Chapter 9

ARTERIAL PULSE PRESSURE


The simulations in the next three chapters are considerably more modest in scope than most of the others in this book. The intent is to illustrate how the graphic capabilities of microcomputers can be used in teaching physical concepts which are basic to the understanding of physiology. This chapter presents a simple physical model which shows how mechanical factors influence the size of the pulsation in the arterial pressure, the "pulse". The computer plots an approximation for the ventricular ejection curve and uses this to compute and plot the arterial pressure for selected values of the important physical parameters.


```
THE MODEL
```

The basis for this model is the classic windkessel model of Otto Frank which dates from the first of this century. This views the arterial system as an elastic container into which the ventricle ejects a stroke volume. The arterial volume and compliance determine the pressure within the compartment. As long as there is any pressure there is a "peripheral runoff" through the systemic vascular beds as determined by a peripheral resistance. Digital solution of the first-order differential equation consists of adding the increments of inflow from the ventricle and subtracting the outflow which goes to the systemic

James E. Randall, Microcomputers and Physiological Simulation

beds. The net volume change during the integration interval
establishes a new volume and a new pressure and the process is
then repeated.

The idea for the present exercise came from a
minicomputer model in a paper by Katz et al (1978). The actual
equations for the model in this chapter are given in BASIC form
in a later section. Figure 9.1 illustrates the major components
which must be appreciated in viewing the computed responses.
The model assumes that the relation between pressure and volume
is linear, i. e., a constant compliance. The peripheral flow is
determined by the pressure and a constant resistance. The
pressure is assumed to rise uniformly throughout the arterial
system so that there is no pulse propagation or wave reflection.
The mathematical function for the ventricular ejection is taken
as the positive half of a sine wave lasting for the duration of
systole. The area under this curve is the stroke volume.
Finally, the aortic valve is assumed to fuction ideally so that
there is no backflow into the ventricle during diastole.

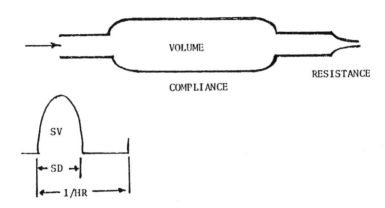

Fig. 9.1. The components of the windkessel model for arterial
    mechanics used in this chapter. Ventricular ejection is a
    sinusoidal function lasting SD seconds out of the total
    cardiac cycle which is the reciprocal of the heart rate HR.
    The area beneath the ejection curve is the stroke volume
    SV. The pressure in the elastic compartment is directly
    proportional to the volume as determined by a constant
    compliance of 1.25 ml/mm Hg. Flow exits according to the
    pressure and a constant resistance of 0.01778 mm Hg/ml/min.
    Either of these parameters may be varied.

In spite of the restrictive nature of these many
assumptions the concept is a standard teaching model in
physiology. The graphic simulation is simply a device to help
visualize that pulse pressure is markedly influenced by stroke

volume and arterial compliance. Greater realism can be achieved
by having the compliance vary as a function of pressure and by
including the option of valvular competence.

---

COMPUTED RESPONSES

---

The accompanying figures are photographs of  simulations
performed  on  the Apple II computer using the program described
in the next section. The output subroutine can be modified  for
other  microcomputers  having  graphic  displays,  but  tabular
solutions are ineffective.      Figure  9.2  shows  the  parameter
selection  and  computed  response for normal circumstances.   In
10-2A the operator has selected the conditions for the exercises
by   answering   the  question  marks  following  the  prompting
questions.   Upon  selecting  the  standard  heart  rate  of  75
beats/min  the  computer  indicates  that  this corresponds to a
cardiac cycle duration of 0.8 sec. This is helpful in the  next
line  which selects the duration of systole. The stroke volume,
aortic  compliance,  and  peripheral  resistance  are  additional
selections.     The   final entry is the initial arterial pressure
which  determines the initial condition for  the  integration  of
the volume as a function of time.

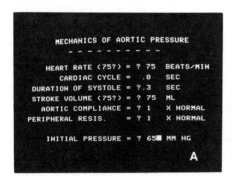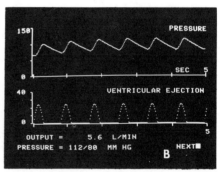

Fig. 9.2.  The selection  of  parameters  (A) and  the  computed
           pressure response (B) for the normal ventricular filling of
           the aorta. The top tracing is in mm Hg; the bottom one  is
           in  liters/min.  The ejection occurs during 0.3 sec of the
           0.8 sec cardiac cycle and delivers a 75 ml  volume  to  the
           artery.    The  cardiac  output  is the product of stroke
           volume and heart rate. The displayed 112/80 mm Hg are  the
           most recent systolic and diastolic values.

Figure 9.2B is a 5-second simulation of the corresponding pressure as computed at 0.02 second increments. The product of heart rate and stroke volume sets the cardiac output as 5,625 ml/min but because ejection occurs only during systole the peak output is over 20 l/min. The pressure started from an initial value of 65 mm Hg and can be seen to rise during the times of ventricular ejection and decay exponentially during diastole. A function of the aortic valve and aortic elasticity is to smooth out the pulsations in pressure which arise from the intermittent nature of the cardiac pumping. The display at the bottom of the figure indicates that the most recent values of systolic and diastolic pressures are 112/80 mm Hg.

There is a gradual rise in arterial pressure during the simulated 5-second period because the initial pressure chosen was slightly below that for the final steady-state conditions. In this model the mean arterial pressure is determined by the cardiac output and the periprheral resistance but the peaks and valleys depend upon other factors.

In the figure it appears as though the pressure excursions do not align vertically with the pulses of blood delivered from the ventricle. One must recall that at the beginning of systole the pressure will not rise until inflow from the ventricle exceeds the ever-present outflow. Thus the pressure upstroke has a shorter duration than the ejection curve does. In addition, the vertical resolution of the pressure tracing is limited to 2 mm Hg per displayed point, a factor which reduces its responsiveness.

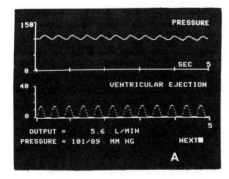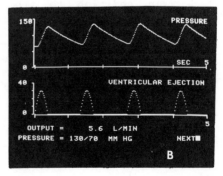

Fig. 9.3. Two simulations in which the cardiac outputs and mean pressures are the same but the pulse pressures differ markedly. In (A) the fast heart rate and low stroke volume give a pulse pressure of only 12 mm Hg. In (B) the slow heart rate and large stroke volume are responsible for the pulse pressure of 60 mm Hg. The mean pressure is 100 units in both cases.

Figure 9.3 shows two simulations where cardiac output is the same in both cases but in which there is a marked difference in pulse pressure. In 9.3A the cardiac output is achieved by a stroke volume of 37.5 ml for a heart rate of 150. The small size of the ejection pulse gives the "fast, weak" pulse. In 9.3B, in which the heart rate is 45 beats/min, the stroke volume of 125 ml is responsible for the large pulse pressure. These conditions are characteristic of persons who are trained physically. Note that the pulse pressure is 12 units for the first case and 60 units in the second. In both simulations the mean pressure is 100 mm Hg as set by the product of cardiac output and the peripheral resistance.

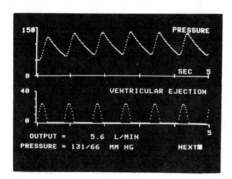

Fig. 9.4. A simulation in which arterial compliance is set to 0.5 times normal. For the standard stroke volume of 75 ml the pulse pressure is now 65 mm Hg. Note that the simulation started from a pressure of 50 units and took several cycles to come to a steady state.

In addition to the stroke volume the rise in arterial pressure depends upon the arterial compliance and upon the rate of ejection during systole. In Figure 9.4 the standard cardiac ouput is achieved by a stroke volume of 75 at a rate of 75 beats/min but the compliance has been reduced to 0.5 normal. Note that the pulse pressure is now 65 even though the stroke volume and mean pressure are the standard values. This simulates a condition of senility in which there is a loss of elasticity but no increase in peripheral resistance. Also, at large arterial pressures the arterial tree becomes less distensible so the pulse pressure increases for these conditions. The compliance itself does not influence the mean arterial pressure unless the peaks of pressure impose an afterload which compromises the ventricular output. It should be emphasized that this simulation assumes constant cardiac output irrespective of the ventricular pressure.

The shorter the time of ejection for a given stroke volume the faster the rate of rise of the pressure. In fact, the rate of change of pressure during systole is a common method of assessing ventricular contractility. Figure 9.5 shows the effects of reducing the duration of systole from 0.3 to 0.2 sec

for a stroke volume of 75 ml. Note that the peak of ejection is
increased to just less than 40 liters/min and that systolic
pressure has risen to 119 mm Hg. If the nonlinear nature of
arterial compliance is included this peaking of the systolic
pressure is even greater.


Fig. 9.5. A simulation in
which the duration of systole
is reduced from 0.3 to 0.2 sec
for a stroke volume of 75 ml.
The elevated ejection rate
raises the systolic pressure
from 112 to 119 mm Hg. Note
that the simulation starts from
a value of 100 units and
gradually falls to a steady
state. The dots on the
ejection tracing are at
increments of 0.02 sec.

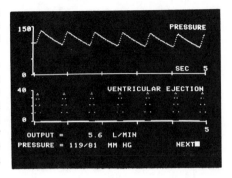

## THE BASIC PROGRAM

        This section describes the essential steps involved in
simulating the graphic displays for arterial pressure. The
Chapter Appendix gives the more complete listing for the program
in Applesoft BASIC except for the routines which place letters
as vectors in the high-resolution graphics area. The modular
plan is given in Table 9.1 as a sequence of subroutine calls
which do specific tasks.

        Line 200 calls the subroutine at line 2000 which asks
for the heart rate, stroke volume and other parameters. Line
400 calls the subroutine which plots the axes using the
high-resolution graphics mode of Applesoft. The iteration loop
is divided into two steps to allow for the differences in
duration and input forcing for the systolic and for the
diastolic intervals. Line 1100 calls the subroutine at line
5000 which computes and displays the ejection function and the
arterial pressure. The subroutine at line 5500, called from
line 1300, differs in that it includes only the diastolic
runoff. The loop is terminated within a display subroutine
called by either the systolic or diastolic computation routines.

```
                          Table 9.1

The  main  routine  for  calling   subroutines   which
establish the physical parameters and then alternately
compute systolic and diastolic intervals of successive
cardiac cycles.


100 REM -- ARTERIAL PULSE PRESSURE MECHANICS --
110 REM     INITIALIZATION
200 :
200 GOSUB 2000          (Get parameters
400 GOSUB 6000          (Hi-resol graph axes
900 :
950 :
1000 REM -- ITERATION LOOP --
1100 GOSUB 5000         (Compute and display systole
1300 GOSUB 5500         (Compute and display diastole
1400 GOTO 1000          (Repeat until display stops it
```

The subroutine at line 2000, given in Table 9.2, assigns
values  to  the parameters used in the computation stages.  This
routine  does  not  include  the  detailed  options,   such   as
formatting lines on the CRT screen, assigning default values, or
detecting out-of-limits entries.  These steps are important  for
successful  use of the computer by students, but their design is
largely a matter of personal taste.

Line 2100 sets the variable T to its initial value.  The
integration interval DT is  set  to  0.02  seconds,  or  0.02/60
minutes,  to  allow  the  250  horizontal  points to represent 5
seconds of time.  This resolution is sufficient for the intended
purposes.   The  variable  HR  is  used for heart rate; SV, for
stroke volume; R, for peripheral resistance; and C, for arterial
compliance.   The  suggested  default value for R is 0.01778 mm
Hg/ml/min to give a mean pressure value of 100  mm  Hg  for  the
cardiac  output which accompanies a stroke volume of 75 ml and a
heart rate of 75 beats/minute.

The  arterial  compliance used was 1.5 ml/mm Hg chosen in
order to give a pulse  pressure  of  about  40  mm  Hg  for  the
indicated  stroke  volume  ejected  within  the typical systolic
interval of 0.3 seconds.  Line 2700 uses the initial pressure to
calculate  the  initial  volume condition for the integration of
the differential equation.  The variables in line 2710 are  used
in  sensing  the systolic and the diastolic pressures during the
iteration process.

```
                        Table 9.2

    Subroutine limited to the essential steps   needed  to
    set  the  physical  parameters of the model. The line
    numbers coordinate with the more detailed  listing  in
    the Chapter Appendix.


    2000  REM  -- GET PARAMETERS --
    2010  TEXT:HOME                     (Clear  screen
    2100  DT = 0.02/60: T = 0: PI = 3.14159
    2200  INPUT "HEART RATE =";HR
    2260  INPUT "SYSTOLE =";SD: SD=SD/60
    2330  INPUT "STROKE VOLUME =";SV
    2410  INPUT "COMPLIANCE =";C
    2460  INPUT "RESISTANCE =";R
    2570  INPUT "INITIAL PRESSURE =";P
    2700  V=P*C
    2710  PD=P: PS=P: P1=P: P2=P
    2800  RETURN
```

        The   reader   is   referred to the Chapter Appendix for the
subroutine at line 6000 which places the axes and tic  marks  on
the Apple II high-resolution graphics display.  The user-defined
labels are omitted.  Line 6100 initializes the graphics area  in
the  mode  which  allows  4  lines  of text at the bottom of the
screen.  Lines 6100-6275 use the HPLOT  X,Y  vector  command  to
place the axes and tic marks as used in the figures in the first
part of this chapter.  Lines 6300-6315 calculate and display the
cardiac output in liters/min keeping only one decimal place

        Table 9.3 contains  the  subroutines  for  the  important
computational steps during systole (lines 5000-5400) and during
diastole (lines 5500-5850).  Line 5100  establishes  a  FOR-NEXT
loop which increments I in steps of the integration interval DT
through the duration of systole SD.  Note  that  I  is  not  an
integer index  but rather a measure of time within the systolic
interval. Line 5150 computes the rate of ventricular  injection
IN at each step during systole.  The quantity (SV/SD) is the
average rate of flow during systole.   But,  this  has  to  be
modified  to  allow  for  the  fact  that  the  flow  changes
sinusoidally during the systolic interval SD.   The  sinusoidal
factor computes the  positive oscillation reaching a peak when
I/SD=0.5.  The term 0.636 is the ratio of  the  average  to  the
peak of a half-cycle of a sine wave and is included to allow for
a peak of IN which is greater than the average (SV/SD).   Line
5200 assures that there  will  be  no  negative  values due to
computational errors.

Table 9.3

Subroutines for computing ventricular ejection during
systole and pressures throughout the cardiac cycle.
In these programs I is not an integer index but rather
the value of time within the systolic or diastolic
intervals. Each of these two subroutines calls a
display subroutine at line 4000 which plots the
variables and determines the end of the simulation.

```
5000 REM -- SYSTOLIC COMPUTATION --
5100 FOR I= 0 TO SD STEP DT
5150    IN = (SV/SD) * SIN(PI*I/SD) / 0.636
5200    IF IN  <  0 THEN IN = 0
5225    GOSUB 4000:REM  PLOT SUBROUTINE
5250    P=V/C: V = V + (IN*DT) - (P*DT/R)
5350    T=T+DT
5360    NEXT I
5400 RETURN
5450 :
5410 :
5500 REM -- DIASTOLIC COMPUTATION --
5600 FOR I= 0 TO (1/HR) - SD  STEP DT
5650    IN = 0
5675    GOSUB 4000: REM  PLOT SUBROUTINE
5700    P=V/C: V = V - (P*DT/R)
5800    T=T+DT
5810    NEXT I
5850 RETURN
```

Line 5225 calls the display subroutine which is
described below.     Line   5250   calculates   the   pressure
corresponding to current arterial volume V and then updates the
volume by Euler integration. The volume is increased during the
integration interval by the product IN*DT. The peripheral
runoff is P/R and that value establishes the loss when
multiplied by the step DT. Line 5350 updates the time variable
used in plotting and then repeats the loop until the end of the
systolic interval.

The subroutine at line 5500 in Table 9.3 applies to the
diastolic interval and contains two major differences. The
stepping of I, established in line 5600, is for the duration of
diastole at steps of DT. Also, unless there is a faulty aortic
value, the injection variable is continually reset as IN=0 in
line 5650. The updating of volume in line 5700 consists of
subtracting out the peripheral runoff during the integration

interval. (For simulation of aortic regurgitation there is an additional factor determined by a valvular resistance that is effective only during diastole.)

```
                            Table 9.4

     Display subroutine for the Apple II microcomputer.
     This plots ventricular ejection and computed pressure
     values and displays the most recent values of systolic
     and diastolic pressure.


     4000 -- PLOT VARIABLES, UPDATE SYSTOLIC/DIASTOLIC --
     4100 X = 25 + 250 * (T * 60/5)          (X= 25 to 275
     4150 Y = 75 - (P/2): IF Y<0 THEN Y=0    (Y=0  top CRT
     4200 HPLOT X,Y                          (Pressure
     4300 HPLOT X,150 - (IN/800)             (Ejection
     4310 :
     4410 IF P1<P2 AND P1<P THEN PD=P1       (Diastolic
     4420 IF P1>P2 AND P1>P THEN PS=P1       (Systolic
     4430 P2=P1: P1=P                        (Keep last 2
     4450 VTAB 24: HTAB 12
     4500 PRINT INT(PS);"/";INT(PD);"  MM HG";
     4800 IF X<275 THEN RETURN               (More x´s
     4820 GET A$: GOTO 100                   (Restart
```

The output subroutine, given in Table 9.4, plots the variables using the HPLOT X,Y command and displays the systolic and diastolic pressures. The origin for the graph is in the upper left corner with a range of 280 horizontal points and 160 vertical points. Line 4100 in the table sets the x-coordinate so that 5 seconds corresponds to the end of the 250-point sweep. The pressure P is plotted above Y=75 as a baseline with a maximum range of 150 mm Hg. Line 4300 plots the ventricular ejection above a baseline of Y=150 and scaled so that each y-ordinate point corresponds to 800 ml/min.

Lines 4410-4430 contain a very simple algorithm for keeping the variable PS set to the most recent systolic pressure and PD set to the diastolic value. Upon each iteration the variable P2 contains the value of P two iterations ago and P1 is set to the value for the previous iteration. P1 is considered a systolic value if it is greater than both P2 and the current P. P1 is considered a diastolic value if it is less than both P2 and P. The balance of this subroutine displays these pressure values at the bottom of the screen. After the x-coordinate reaches a value of 275 at the left edge the program waits for a key to be pressed to restart the simulation.

REFERENCES

Beeuwkes. R., and N. Braslow: The cardiovascular analog trainer:
A real time physiological simulator. Physiol. Teacher. 3:4-7
(1974).

Brubakk, A. O., and R. Aaslid: Use of a model for simulating
individual aortic dynamics in man. Med. & Biol. Eng. & Comput.
16:231-242 (1978).

Green, J. F. Mechanical Concepts in Cardiovascular and Pulmonary
Physiology. Philadelphia: Lea & Febiger (1977)

Katz, S., R. G. Hollingsworth, J. G. Blackburn, and H. T.
Carter:    Computer    simulation   in   the   physiology  student
laboratory.   Physiol. Teacher,  Physiologist 45:41-44 (1978).

CHAPTER APPENDIX

        The following listing is  the  Applesoft  BASIC  routine
which produces the displays in the figures of this chapter.  The
routines    which    place    labels    as    vectors   within    the
high-resolution  graphics  area  are   not   included.    The axes
subroutine at line 6000 and the plot  subroutine   at   line   4000
must be changed to run this program on other microcomputers.

```
10    REM    PLOTS VENTRICULAR EJECTION AND ARTERIAL PRESSURE
20    REM    PARAMETERS: HEART RATE, SYSTOLE DURATION, STROKE VOLUME
30    REM      ARTERIAL COMPLIANCE, PERIPHERAL RESISTANCE
40    REM    DISPLAYS CARDIAC OUTPUT
50    REM      AND SYSTOLIC/DIASTOLIC PRESSURES
60  :
70  :
100   REM   --> INITIALIZATION <--
200   GOSUB 2000: REM    GET PARAMETERS
400   GOSUB 6000: REM    PLOT AXES
900  :
950  :
1000   REM    -- ITERATION LOOP <-----
1100   GOSUB 5000: REM   SYSTOLE
1300   GOSUB 5500: REM   DIASTOLE
1500   GOTO 1000: REM    ------------>
1700  :
1800  :
1900  :
2000   REM   --> GET PARAMETERS <--
2010   TEXT : HOME
2020   HTAB 7: PRINT "MECHANICS OF AORTIC PRESSURE"
2025   VTAB 3
2030   HTAB 10: PRINT "- - - - - - - - - - "
2100  DT = .02 / 60:T = 0:PI = 3.14159
2195   VTAB 6: HTAB 5
2200   INPUT "HEART RATE (75?) = ? ";HR
2210   VTAB 6: HTAB 30: PRINT "BEATS/MIN";
2215   VTAB 8: HTAB 8
2220   PRINT "CARDIAC CYCLE =  "; INT (6000 / HR) / 100;
2225   HTAB 30: PRINT "SEC";
2250   VTAB 10: HTAB 2
2260   INPUT "DURATION OF SYSTOLE = ?";SD:SD = SD / 60
2270   VTAB 10: HTAB 30: PRINT "SEC";
2320   VTAB 12: HTAB 2
2330   INPUT "STROKE VOLUME (75?) = ?";SV
2340   VTAB 12: HTAB 30: PRINT "ML"
2400   PRINT
2410   HTAB 4: INPUT "AORTIC COMPLIANCE = ?";C
2420  C = C * 1.25
2430   VTAB 14: HTAB 30: PRINT "X NORMAL"
2450   PRINT
2460   HTAB 1: INPUT "PERIPHERAL RESIS.    = ?";R
2470  R = R * 0.01778
2480   VTAB 16: HTAB 30: PRINT "X NORMAL"
2560   VTAB 20: HTAB 5
2570   INPUT "INITIAL PRESSURE = ?";P
2580   VTAB 20: HTAB 30: PRINT "MM HG"
2700  V = P * C
2710  PD = P:PS = P:P1 = P:P2 = P
2800   RETURN
```

```
4000   REM  --> PLOT VARIABLES <--
4100 X = 25 + 250 * (T * 60 / 5)
4150 Y = 75 - (P / 2): IF Y < 0 THEN Y = 0
4200   HPLOT X,Y
4300   HPLOT X,150 - (IN / 800)
4410   IF Pl < P2 AND Pl < P THEN PD = Pl
4420   IF Pl > P2 AND Pl > P THEN PS = Pl
4430 P2 = Pl:Pl = P
4450   VTAB 24: HTAB 12
4500   PRINT  INT (PS);"/"; INT (PD);" ";
4510   HTAB 20: PRINT "MM HG";
4800   IF X = < 275 THEN  RETURN
4810   VTAB 24: HTAB 40: GET A$: GOTO 100
4998 :
4999 :
5000   REM  --> SYSTOLE COMPUTATIONS <--
5100   FOR I = 0 TO SD STEP DT
5150 IN = (SV / SD) *  SIN (PI * I / SD) / .636
5200   IF IN < 0 THEN IN = 0
5225   GOSUB 4000: REM    PLOT VARIABLES
5250 P = V / C:V = V + (IN * DT) - (P * DT / R)
5350 T = T + DT: NEXT I
5400   RETURN
5450 :
5460 :
5500   REM  --> DIASTOLE COMPUTATIONS <--
5600   FOR I = 0 TO (1 / HR) - SD STEP DT
5650 IN = 0: GOSUB 4000: REM    PLOT VARIBLES
5700 P = V / C:V = V - (P / R) * DT
5800 T = T + DT: NEXT I
5850   RETURN
5998 :
5999 :
6000   REM  --> PLOT AXES AND LABELS <--
6100   HGR : HPLOT 25,75 TO 275,75: HPLOT 25,151 TO 275,151
6150   FOR Xl = 25 TO 275 STEP 50: HPLOT Xl,72 TO Xl,77
6160   HPLOT Xl,155 TO Xl,152: NEXT Xl
6200   HPLOT 19,0 TO 19,75: HPLOT 19,100 TO 19,150
6225   FOR Yl = 0 TO 75 STEP 25
6230   HPLOT 17,Yl TO 18,Yl: NEXT Yl
6250   FOR Yl = 100 TO 150 STEP 12.5
6275   HPLOT 17,Yl TO 18,Yl: NEXT Yl
6300   VTAB 22: HTAB 1: PRINT "  OUTPUT = ";
6305   HTAB 16: PRINT  INT (HR * SV / 100) / 10;
6315   HTAB 20: PRINT "L/MIN";
6360   HTAB 1: VTAB 24: PRINT "PRESSURE = ";
6900   RETURN
```

Chapter 10

VECTORCARDIOGRAPHY AND THE LIMB LEADS


The exercise in this chapter is modest in scope but chosen to illustrate how interactive graphics can provide effective lecture deomonstrations. The microcomputer program plots the deflections in the three electrocadiogram limb leads as components of a single equivalent vector, a concept which is a basic tenet of introductory electrocardiography.

The vectorcardiogram is used clinically as a method for rapid visualization of the instantaneous direction of the mean direction of electrical currents during ventricular excitation. Shifts of the mean electrical axis can be correlated with the anatomical postion of the heart, as with the horizontal displacement during pregnancy, or with prolonged conduction, as with ventricular hypertrophy. In addition, the loop described by the successive vectors during ventricular depolarization, provides a rational basis for the relative magnitudes and directions of the deflections in the three limb leads.

The exercise in this chapter permits a student to pick an angle for the mean electrical axis of the ventricular depolarization and then the computer displays both the QRS vector loop and its components as projections onto the axes of the three limb leads, I, II, and III. The display dynamically illustrates the correlation between the temporal sequence of points on the vectorcardiogram and their scalar components. It provides a wide range of illustrations of relative deflections in the leads each showing that the deflection in Leads I and III sum to that in lead II at any one instant in time.

James E. Randall, Microcomputers and Physiological Simulation

The basic assumption for the model in its simplest form is that the body-surface potential differences, as measured in leads I, II, and III, are equivalent to those that might be expected if the heart were to be replaced by a single equivalent dipole which changed in magnitude and direction during cardiac excitation and repolarization. Furthermore, the axes of these three leads are assumed to be spaced at equal angles of 60 degrees each.    Thus the deflection in lead I is assumed to be the horizontal component of the dipole's vector representation at any instant. Lead II's axis is considered along the axis of the heart, that is, from right arm to left leg.    The axis of lead III bisects the angle between the axes of the other two.

It must be emphasized that this representation is a very simple one, meant for beginning students in physiology.  There are many elaborate methods of localizing electrode placements to try to achieve true orthogonality of the vector axes in the anterior-posterior plane as well as in the frontal plane.    In addition, the concept of the heart as a single equivalent dipole is unsatisfactory for many pathological circumstances and for potentials measured near the heart.

The computer program presented reduces the concept to its simplest form as an illustration of what can be done with graphic displays in microcomputers. The program has a stored table of 20 pairs of scaled x- and y-coordinates for the vector at equal time intervals during ventricular excitation.  The mean axis of the loop described by the ends of these vectors lies along the line of lead II, at 60 degrees below the horizontal. The student picks an angle by which the axis of the loop is to be deviated from normal, negative values corresponding to left-axis deviations.    The program rotates the angle of each vector by the indicated amount and plots their corresponding tips superimposed on the axes of the limb leads. At the same time the scalar projections upon these axes are plotted as scalar functions of time.    The program could be expanded to include a variety of differently shaped loops,      the anterior-posterior component, and the atrial depolarization and ventricular repolarization parts of the total cardiac cycle.

The program given is written in Applesoft BASIC but it uses certain generalized features for ease of transcription to other graphic displays. It includes a special numerical device to simulate the fact that the vector loop is generally counterclockwise for left-axis deviations. The angle at which the direction of the loop is reversed is arbitrarily chosen, as is the range for classification for a "normal" mean electrical axis. Many of the program's unessential steps are eliminated from discussion in the text but a complete Applesoft listing is given in the Chapter Appendix.

COMPUTED RESPONSES

The responses in the accompanying figures are photographs of Apple II CRT displays for three different angles of the axis of the stored oval-shaped vectorcardiogram loop. In practice extreme deviations of the QRS loop's mean direction are likely to be accompanied by complex patterns of the loop itself, so students must continually be reminded of the restraints of the model. It is not uncommon to see loops of the form given here for a modest range of mean electrical axes. Figure 10.1 shows the instructions and computed response for simulating a normal vectorcardiogram which lies along lead II. In A) the student has supplied a value of "0" degrees as the deviation from normal. The cursor is waiting for the operator to press the return key to proceed with the computation and display as given in B).

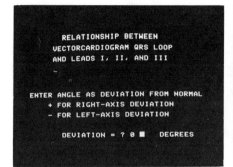 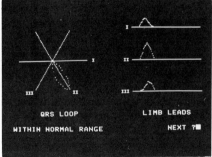

Fig. 10.1. Selection of the axis of the vectorgram loop A) and its display along with the corresponding deflections in the three limb leads B). The angle of the loop is entered as a deviation from normal. The three scalar leads are plotted at one-half scale of their vector projections onto their respective axes. The vectorcardiogram consists of 20 data pairs stored in a table.

The axes and label require only a few seconds to be displayed. The total time for plotting the vector loop and the deflections in I, II, and III also takes only a few seconds, but it easily could be slowed down in order to allow time for appreciation of the temporal sequence and relationship between the different tracings. When these are finished the bottom line indicates the classification of the deviation and waits for a keyboard response to proceed with the next simulation.

   The loop in Figure 10.1B is plotted in a clockwise
direction and as each dot is placed on the triaxial display the
corresponding  components  are  plotted at one-half scale on the
three limb leads at the right of the figure.   It can be seen
that  the  amplitude  of  lead II  is  largest  and  that  the
deflections in leads I and III are about equal corresponding  to
the  projections  of  the vectors onto these axes.  Furthermore,
the instantaneous deflections in I and in III sum  to  those  in
II.

   In Figure 10.2 the angle  chosen  is  -65  degrees  from
normal and is classified as a left-axis deviation.   In this case
the loop is plotted counterclockwise, corresponding to the  fact
that  during the initial parts of ventricular depolarization the
direction of the vector  is  generally  toward  the  lower  left
quadrant.    The  axis of this loop is very nearly horizontal so
that lead I has a large upright deflection.  The projection onto
lead III is such that it has a downward deflection corresponding
to the fact that the left leg is negative with  respect  to  the
left  arm.   Lead II in this case is small.  Note again that the
deflections in Leads I and III sum to those in lead II.

Figure  10.2.  Vectorcardiogram
QRS  loop  and  corresponding
three  limb  leads  for an angle
of  -65  degrees.    This  is
classified  as  a  left-axis
deviation  which  has  a  large
deflection  in  lead  I  and  a
downward one in lead III.

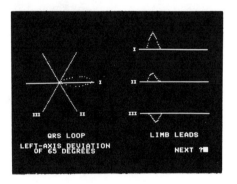

   In  Figure  10.3  the  chosen  angle  is  90  degrees
corresponding to an extreme right-axis deviation.  The  dots  in
the  loop are plotted clockwise as time progresses and lie along
a line between the axes of lead III  and  the  side  of  lead  I
corresponding  to  downward  deflections  in that lead.  Note the
large upright deflection in Lead I and the downward one  in  III
so  that  their sum gives the very small lead II.  This angle is
chosen to illustrate a biphasic response in II  where  it  first
has  an  R wave  at  the time that the vector projects onto the
positive half of lead II's axis.

   Before leaving this section it should be said once again
that the purpose of this exercise is limited to illustrating the
direction  and  relative  magnitudes  of  the deflections in the
three  limb  leads  for  shifts  in  the  direction  of  the  mean

electrical axis during ventricular depolarization. This can be
a helpful exercise to the beginning student but it should not be
used to infer more than this simple concept.  For   realism   the
shape   of  the loop should be a parameter and perhaps a function
of extreme amounts of shift of the mean axis.

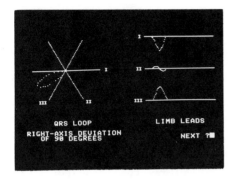

Figure   10.3.    QRS   loop   of
vectorcardiogram  and  limb-lead
deflections   for   a  right-axis
deviation  of  90  degrees   from
the  normal  value.   Note  the
small  biphasic  deflection   in
lead  II  corresponding  to  the
fact  that  the  loop's  direction
is  perpendicular   to  the  axis
of that lead.

---

THE BASIC PROGRAM

---

        This section presents the main features of an  Applesoft
BASIC  program  which  computes  and  plots the vectorcardiogram
loops and scalar deflections  for  chosen  angles  of  the  mean
electrical  axis.   At an increase in complexity of notation the
program uses generalized origins for the  axes  and  a  vertical
scale  factor  to  allow  adaptation  to  other  graphic display
formats. The  program  requires  a  modest  amount  of  graphic
resolution  and  is not apt to be effective on graphs plotted by
alphanumeric characters in columns and rows.

        Table  10.1  presents  the  main  routine  which  calls a
series of modular subroutines.   Lines  1000-1030  set  up  the
parameters  and  vector  array, lines 1050-1130 are executed for
each new chosen angle of the vector loop.  Line  1010  dimensions
two  arrays  which can contain up to 25 pairs of coordinates for
the stored vector loop.  The subroutine at line 1500 establishes
factors  for  converting  between degrees and radians.  Line 1540
sets the origin for the vector loop at X0=60 and  Y=80  for  the
Apple microcomputer, but different values may be appropriate for
other graphic displays.

        The  Apple  high-resolution  graphics mode requires that
y-deflections be multiplied by a factor of FA=1.05 in  order  to
give  equal scales for vertical and horizontal deflections. This
factor must equal 1.7 for the Matrox  CRT  interface  used  with
S-100 bus microcomputers and described in Chapter 4.  Line  1560

uses X1,Y1 as the origin for the temporal plot of lead I and Y2 and Y3 as the ordinates for leads II and III respectively.

In Table 10.1 line 1060 calls the subroutine at line 5000. The essense of this subroutine, contained in the full listing at the end of the chapter, is to ask the user for the desired angle by which to rotate the vectorcardiogram loop from normal. This consists of the statement

        5100 INPUT "DEVIATION = "; ANG.

Line 1070 calls the routine at line 6000 which plots the axes and labels using the high-resolution graphics mode.

---

Table 10.1

Main routine which calls subroutines to initialize parameters and to compute and display the tracings. The subroutine at lines 1500-1570 establishes the origins on the display for these tracings according to the graphics of the microcomputer being used.

```
1000 REM -- INITIALIZATION --
1010 CLEAR: DIM X(25),Y(25)
1020 GOSUB 1500                    (Set parameters
1030 GOSUB 2000                    (Move corrdinates
1040:
1050 REM   EACH NEW QRS LOOP <-------
1060 GOSUB 5000                    (Title, get angle
1070 GOSUB 6000                    (Axes, labels
1080 IF ANG<-10 THEN K=21: L=-1    (CCW loop
1090 IF ANG=>10 THEN K=0:  L=1     (CW loop
1100 GOSUB 3000                    (Loop and leads
1110 GOSUB 7000                    (Bottom line
1130 GET A$: GOTO 1060 ----------->
1140:
1500 REM -- SET UP PARAMETERS --
1520 DE=360/(2*3.1415926): RA = 1/DE
1540 X0=60: Y0=80: FA=1.05         (Origin, DY/DX
1560 X1=175: Y1=30: Y2=80: Y3=130  (Lead origins
1570 RETURN
```

---

Lines 1080 and 1090 set two parameters depending upon the angle chosen for the loop. The purpose of this is to add realism to the temporal sequence of the directions of the vectors. This is necessary because the common finding is that at the start of ventricular depolarization the direction of the mean electrical axis is generally toward the lower left quadrant. For extreme left-axis deviation it then shifts counterclockwise, as viewed on the display device, corresponding to the later depolarization of the left venctricular mass, for example. For right-axis deviation, as with enlarged right ventricular mass, the vector rotates clockwise.

In order to have one set of stored vectors handle both situations the program picks parameters K and L according to the angle of the vector loop. For clockwise rotation the vectors are used in the order stored in the table; for counterclockwise rotation they are called in reverse order from the table. The dividing line between the two cases was rather arbitrarily chosen at -10 degrees.

Once the angle of the vector loop and its direction are chosen the routine at line 3000 computes and displays the loop and the limb-lead deflections. Lines 1110-1130 classify the degree of rotation and wait for a key to be struck to restart with the next selected angle.

---

Table 10.2

Subroutine which moves 20 pairs of vector components into the arrays X(I) and Y(I). The values given are scaled down from a single electrocardiogram QRS tracing. The size of these arrays could be increased for greater resolution and to include the T-wave repolarization part of the process.


```
2000 REM -- PUT 20 DATA PAIRS INTO ARRAYS --
2010 RESTORE: FOR I = 1 TO 20: READ X(I), Y(I): NEXT
2020 RETURN
2030 DATA 03,02, 07,05, 10,08, 12,11, 15,15
2040 DATA 20,24, 22,27, 23,31, 23,34, 24,38
2050 DATA 21,43, 18,42, 15,39, 13,36, 10,33
2060 DATA 07,29, 05,25, 02,17, 01,11, 01,05
2070:
```

---

Let us now exam the key steps in some detail. Table 10.2 contains the subroutine which moves the vector components into arrays from which they are used as subscripted variables. Lines 2030-2060 are BASIC DATA statements containing 20 pairs of x- and y-coordinates for successive values of the ventricular excitation vector. These are scaled from their original measurements for convenience of manual entry into the program. Line 2010 moves these into two arrays with X(I) being the horizontal component and Y(I) the corresponding vertical component. These values can be extended in variety for different clinical loops and in size to include the P and S-T parts of the electrocardiogram.

---

### Table 10.3

Subroutine which plots and displays rotated vector loop and the three limb-lead components. The parameters K and L determine the order of taking the vectors from the table and thus the direction of rotation of the vector loop for increasing time. ANG is the angle of rotation and TH is the final angle of the vectors as displayed. V is the length of the vector. FA is a scaling factor chosen to make vertical increments display the same size as do the horizontal ones.

```
3000 REM -- VECTOR & SCALAR CALCULATIONS AND PLOTS --
3010 FOR I = 1 TO 20: J = K + L*I
3020    V = SQR(X(J)*X(J) + X(J)*X(J))
3030    TH = RA * ANG + ATN(Y(J)/X(J))
3040    HPLOT X0 + V*COS(TH), Y0 + FA*V*SIN(TH)
3050    V=V/2
3080    HPLOT X1+10+I, Y1 - FA*V*COS(TH)
3090    HPLOT X1+10+I, Y2 - FA*V*COS(RA*60-TH)
3100    HPLOT X1+10+I, Y3 - FA*V*COS(RA*120-TH)
3110 NEXT I
```

---

The computation and display subroutine is in lines 3000-3120, given in Table 10.3. Line 3010 starts a FOR-NEXT loop in which the index I corresponds to the successive elements in the vector loop, 20 being the total number in this program. The index J determines where the vector comes from in the table. It starts from the first of the table for clockwise loops but works from the last to first entries for the counterclockwise loops characteristic of left-axis deviation. Line 3020 sets the variable V to the length of the current vector. Line 3030 defines the angle of the rotated vector TH(eta) as the sum of the angle of the vector in the table and the angle selected for the rotation of the total loop. This is given in radians to correspond with the notation used in the BASIC cosine and sine functions.

Line 3040 plots each rotated vector's tip as an offset from the origin defined at X0,Y0. The horizontal deflection is V*COS(TH) and the vertical deflection is V*FA*SIN(TH). The factor FA is necessary because the dot spacing for horizontal and vertical displacements may not be the same. The three limb-lead deflections are plotted in lines 3080-3100 as vector projections at angles of 0, 60, and 120 degrees.

The full subroutine for plotting the axes and their labels is given at the end of the chapter. One aspect does need special mention and is given in Table 10.4. When the slanting axes for leads II and III are drawn using HPLOT vector commands the lines are coarse because the algorithm used fills in more than one y-value at each x-value. The author found it more eye-pleasing to generate the lines by the algorithm in lines 6070-6100 which place one value of y at each value of x. To achieve a 60-degree slope on the CRT the computed increment of y must be FA*1.732. These two lines have YU (up) and YD (down) for their origins.

---

Table 10.4

Routine to draw the axes of leads II and III at 60 degrees through their origin X0,Y0. In contrast to a HPLOT vector command this algorithm has only one y-value at each x-value.

```
6055 REM -- DRAW AXES FOR II AND III AT 60 DEGREES --
6060 YU = Y0 - 25 * FA * 1.732
6065 YD = Y0 + 25 * FA * 1.732
6070 FOR I= 0 TO 50: XI = X0 - 25 + I
6080   HPLOT XI, YU + I * FA * 1.732
6090   HPLOT XI, YD - I * FA * 1.732
6100 NEXT I
```

---

CHAPTER APPENDIX

Listing of the Applesoft BASIC program which plots vectorcardiogram loops and the three limb leads for selected rotations of the electrical axis. The routine at lines 6120-6530 place the labels using the HPLOT command. Text is placed in the bottom four lines of the first page of the Apple II high-resolution graphics area.

```
100   REM    --- COMPONENTS OF VECTORCARDIOGRAM ---
110   REM        APPLESOFT LISTING FOR APPLE II
120 :
1000  REM    --- INITIALIZATION ---
1010  CLEAR : DIM X(25),Y(25)
1020  GOSUB 1500: REM    SET PARAMETERS
1030  GOSUB 2000: REM    COORDINATES INTO ARRAY
1040 :
1050 : REM    EACH NEW QRS LOOP <-----------
1060  GOSUB 5000: REM    TITLE, GET DEVIATION
1070  GOSUB 6000: REM    AXES AND LABELS
1080  IF ANG < - 10 THEN K = 21:L = - 1: REM    CCW LOOP
1090  IF ANG = > - 10 THEN K = 0:L = 1: REM    CW LOOP
1100  GOSUB 3000: REM    LOOP AND LEADS
1110  GOSUB 7000: REM    PRINT BOTTOM LINE
1120  HTAB 33: VTAB 24: PRINT "NEXT ?";
1130  GET A$: GOTO 1060: REM --REPEAT----->
1140 :
1150 :
1500  REM    --- SET UP PARAMETERS ---
1520 DE = 360 / (2 * 3.1415926):RA = 1 / DE
1530  REM  AXES ORIGINS, FA(CTOR)=CRT DY/DX
1540 X0 = 60:Y0 = 80:FA = 1.05
1550  REM  SCALAR AXES ORIGINS
1560 X1 = 175:Y1 = 30:Y2 = 80:Y3 = 130
1570  RETURN
1580 :
1590 :
2000  REM    --- PUT 20 DATA PAIRS INTO ARRAYS ---
2010  RESTORE : FOR I = 1 TO 20: READ X(I): READ Y(I): NEXT
2020  RETURN
2030  DATA   03,02, 07,05, 10,08, 12,11, 15,15
2040  DATA   20,24, 22,27, 23,31, 23,34, 24,38
2050  DATA   21,43, 18,42, 15,39, 13,36, 10,33
2060  DATA   07,29, 05,25, 02,17, 01,11, 01,05
2070 :
2080 :
3000  REM    --- VECTOR & SCALAR CALCULATIONS AND PLOTS ---
3010  FOR I = 1 TO 20:J = K + L * I
3020 V =  SQR (X(J) * X(J) + Y(J) * Y(J))
3030 TH = RA * ANG +  ATN (Y(J) / X(J))
3040  HPLOT X0 + V *  COS (TH),Y0 + FA * V *  SIN (TH)
3050 V = V / 2
3060 Y = Y1 - FA * V *  COS (TH)
3070  IF Y < 0 THEN Y = 0
3080  HPLOT X1 + 10 + I,Y
3090  HPLOT X1 + 10 + I,Y2 - FA * V *  COS (RA * 60 - TH)
3100  HPLOT X1 + 10 + I,Y3 - FA * V *  COS (RA * 120 - TH)
3110  NEXT I
3120  RETURN
```

```
5000    REM     --- TITLE AND PICK ANGLE ---
5010    TEXT : HOME
5020    HTAB 10: VTAB 1: PRINT "RELATIONSHIP BETWEEN"
5030    HTAB 7: VTAB 3: PRINT " VECTORCARDIOGRAM QRS LOOP"
5040    HTAB 8: VTAB 5: PRINT "AND LEADS I, II, AND III"
5050    HTAB 3: VTAB 12
5060    PRINT "ENTER ANGLE AS DEVIATION FROM NORMAL"
5070    HTAB 7: VTAB 14: PRINT "+ FOR RIGHT-AXIS DEVIATION";
5080    HTAB 7: VTAB 16: PRINT "- FOR LEFT-AXIS DEVIATION";
5090    HTAB 30: VTAB 20: PRINT "DEGREES"
5100    HTAB 10: VTAB 20: INPUT "DEVIATION = ?";ANG
5110    RETURN
5120    :
6000    REM     --- AXES AND LABELS ---
6010    HGR
6020    HPLOT X0 - 50,Y0 TO X0 + 50,Y0
6030    HPLOT X1,Y1 TO X1 + 100,Y1
6040    HPLOT X1,Y2 TO X1 + 100,Y2
6050    HPLOT X1,Y3 TO X1 + 100,Y3
6060    YU = Y0 - 25 * FA * 1.732:YD = Y0 + 25 * FA * 1.732
6070    FOR I = 0 TO 50:XI = X0 - 25 + I
6080    HPLOT XI,YU + I * FA * 1.732
6090    HPLOT XI,YD - I * FA * 1.732
6100    NEXT I
6110    :
6120    XX = X0 + 58:YY = Y0 - 2: GOSUB 6500
6130    XX = 90:YY = 128: GOSUB 6500
6140    XX = XX + 4: GOSUB 6500
6150    XX = 20: GOSUB 6500:XX = XX + 4: GOSUB 6500
6160    XX = XX + 4: GOSUB 6500
6170    XX = X1 - 8:YY = Y1 - 2: GOSUB 6500
6180    XX = X1 - 12:YY = Y2 - 2: GOSUB 6500
6190    XX = XX + 4: GOSUB 6500
6200    XX = X1 - 16:YY = Y3 - 2: GOSUB 6500
6210    XX = XX + 4: GOSUB 6500
6220    XX = XX + 4: GOSUB 6500: RETURN
6270    :
6500     HPLOT XX,YY TO XX + 2,YY
6510     HPLOT XX + 1,YY + 1 TO XX + 1,YY + 3
6520     HPLOT XX,YY + 4 TO XX + 2,YY + 4
6530     RETURN
6540    :
7000    REM     --- DEVIATION ON BOTTOM LINE ---
7010    IF ANG < 0 THEN A$ = "LEFT-AXIS DEVIATION"
7020    IF AN > 45 OR AN < - 45 THEN  GOTO 7040
7030    HTAB 1: VTAB 24: PRINT "WITHIN NORMAL RANGE";: RETURN
7040    IF ANG > 0 THEN A$ = "RIGHT-AXIS DEVIATION"
7050    HTAB 1: VTAB 23: PRINT A$;
7060    HTAB 1: VTAB 24: PRINT "   OF ";
7070    PRINT  ABS ( INT (ANG));" DEGREES";
7080    RETURN
```

Chapter 11

DISTORTION OF WAVEFORMS


When dynamic physiological variables are recorded for study and publication the characteristics of the recording instrument may distort the true waveforms. Often the recorder's characteristics can be quantified by a single parameter, its "time constant". The simulation in this chapter permits visualization of true and distorted waveforms for three dynamic signals and for arbitrarily chosen time constants. It illustrates, for example, the expected arterial pressure and ECG tracings for different degrees of filtering as selected by switch settings on laboratory strip-chart recorders. These filters are used to reduce the noise in laboratory recordings of the electrocardiogram and the exercise shows the consequent distortion produced by the filtering process. When arterial pressures are recorded using time constants having magnitudes of the order of seconds the tracing can be used as a running estimate of the mean pressures.

The implications of the simulations can be extended for the more serious students of physiological instrumentation. The mathematical model for the filtering process is a first-order differential equation having the physiological variable as the input forcing and the filtered output as the solution to the differential equation. One input option is a sinusoidal wave of arbitrarily chosen frequency. The simulations recursively compute the output, a solution which could be obtained analytically. The choice of different frequencies and time

James E. Randall, Microcomputers and Physiological Simulation

constants  allows   a   student   to   gain   appreciation   of   the
"frequency domain" transformations for first-order processes  in
general.  In addition, the simulation shows the power of digital
solutions  for  differential  equations  in  which  the  forcing
functions cannot be represented by analytical expressions.

        Finally, the chapter illustrates digital filtering,  a
process  which  transforms  a  sequence  of  input samples into a
sequence of output values in order to modify selected  frequency
components  in  the sampled waveform.  For a filter which can be
represented by a first-order differential equation each  output
value   is   computed  from  the  present  input  value  and  the
preceeding output, an operation  which  can  be  performed  very
rapidly.   Furthermore,  this  method is not subject to certain
errors inherent in  sampling  a  continuous  process  at  finite
increments of time.

        A teaching exercise is suggested in which the student is
given   the   choice   of   three   different  kinds  of  waveforms:
sinusoidal oscillations of different frequencies,   2.5  seconds
of  an  arterial pressure tracing, and a tracing of an ECG.  The
student then can enter a time constant and see a display of  the
computed   output   for   that   degree  of  filtering.   These
illustrations are followed by a discussion of the simplicity  of
designing   and   programming   first-order   "autoregressive"
processes.  The Chapter Appendix contains the Apple  II  listing
of  the program which produces the figures in this chapter.  The
digitized samples of the pressure and ECG waveforms  are  stored
as  data statements in that program.  One section of the chapter
describes the essential features of the listed program.


        ┌──────────────────────────┐
        │  COMPUTED RESPONSES      │
        └──────────────────────────┘


        The accompanying figures illustrate  how  microcomputers
are  used  to  demonstrate dynamic phenomena through interactive
graphics.  When the program is  started,  digitized  samples  of
waveforms  are  read  into  an array in memory where they can be
accessed rapidly, but a much wider range of  tracings  could  be
stored  on  a  disk.   The  first-order filter was chosen for
simplicity, but this could be extended  to  include  second-  or
higher-order  models  with  additional  programming.   Also, the
display formats used here are  designed  for  one  microcomputer
having graphics capabilities integrated into the BASIC commands.
Tabular solutions are possible, but these are  not  particularly
effective for the purposes of the simulations.

        Figure 11.1A shows the text display from which a  student
selects  the  sinusoidal  waveform to be filtered.  In this case
the first option, for a sinusoidal wave, is chosen.  The program

acknowledges this and requests the frequency of the oscillation,
suggesting values of less than 5 Hz. Once this parameter is
entered the display switches to the graphics mode and plots out
a 2.5-second tracing at the selected frequency, such as the
larger 0.8 Hz oscillation shown in Figure 11.1B. When this is
completed the program requests a numerical value for the time
constant and then computes and displays the appropriate
response.

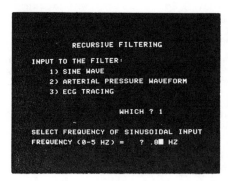 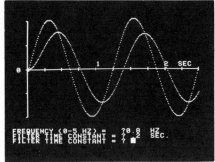

Fig. 11.1. A) Picking the sinuosidal input option and selecting
a frequency. B) Display of a 2.5-second segment of a 0.8
Hz oscillation and the computed response for a 0.2-second
time constant. The amplitude of the output oscillation is
70.7% of that of the input and it also lags the input by 45
degrees.


In the figure a time constant of 0.2 second is specified
because that value corresponds to the reciprocal of the input
frequency when expressed as 5 radians/sec. At this reciprocal
combination of frequency and time constant the output signal has
an amplitude which is 0.707 times the input and the output lags
1/8 cycle behind the input forcing. This is apparent in the
simulation given in the figure. Also note that since the
solution starts from a first value of zero, there is an initial
transient before the output falls into a steady-state condition
where each point is exactly 1/8 cycle behind the input.

As a further illustration of the frequency-dependence
of first-order processes Figure 11.2 shows an input waveform at
2.4 Hz and the computed response for a time constant of 0.2
seconds, the same as used in the previous illustration. This
shows that as the frequency of the forcing increases the
response is reduced in amplitude and delayed in time. When the
frequency, expressed in radians per second, is greater than 50
times the time constant the output becomes undetectable at the
resolution of the display. Such a filter is called "low-pass"

Figure 11.2. Simulation of computed response of a first-order process having a time constant of 0.2 second but driven by an oscillation of 2.4 Hz. Note the reduction in output and increase in phase lag as compared to that in the previous figure. This is characteristic of instruments which act like "low-pass" filters.

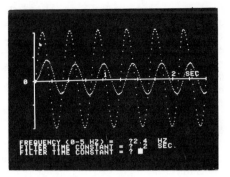

because it attenuates the high-frequency components more than it does the low-frequency ones. Conversely, a whole family of output waveforms can be plotted at different time constants superimposed upon the same input tracing to illustrate the effects of changing this characteristic of a recording instrument.

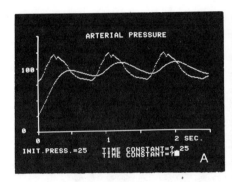

Fig. 11.3. Computed responses for arterial pressure waveforms as measured with instruments characterized by time constants of a first-order process. A) shows the response starting from 25 mm Hg and a time constant of .25 seconds, a value which retains some of the features of the normal cardiac cycle fluctuations, though reduced in amplitude and lagging in phase. The response in B) is for a time constant of 2 seconds so that the tracing is severely distorted but it does indicate the mean pressure.

When pressure is chosen as the input to the filter, samples taken at 0.01-second intervals are displayed on the screen, as shown by the large oscillations in Figure 11.3. The

computer asks for an initial pressure and a time constant and
uses these values to compute and display the response. In A) of
this figure the solution is started from 25 mm Hg with a time
constant of 0.25 seconds. Note that there is an initial
transient before the filtered output falls into step lagging
behind the true pressure. At this time constant the
high-frequency dicrotic notch is filtered out but the pressure
follows the cardiac pulsations, though with reduced amplitude
and with a lagging of the peaks and valleys of the pulse
pressure.

In B) of this figure the time constant is increased to 2
seconds and the solution starts at 90 mm Hg which is near the
steady-state value. The waveform is severely distorted but is a
measure of the mean arterial pressure.

The final illustration, Figure 11.4, shows computed
responses when the input is an electrocardiogram. In A) the
filtering has a parameter of 0.02 seconds, one short enough to
retain the time of the R deflection, but reducing its amplitude
significantly. Note that the slower P and T waves are not
modified to any great extent.

In B), the time constant has the much longer value of
0.1 seconds, the distortion is even greater. It is possible to
superimpose several solutions at different time constants,
though these can become too cluttered to be useful. The program
has the option of restarting if no value is entered in the
response to a query.

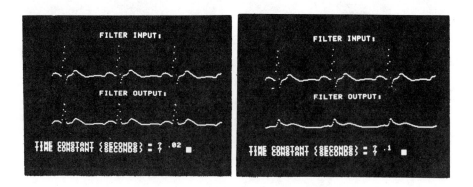

Fig. 11.4. Computed responses for electrocardiograms recorded
    by first-order instruments with different time constants.
    A) has a time constant of 0.02 seconds and attentuates the
    fast R and S waves, with little influence upon the slower P
    and T waves. B) has a time constant of 0.1 seconds, a time
    comparable to the duration of the QRS complex so that this
    is markedly reduced.

> DIGITAL FILTERING

The defining differential equation for the first-order filter is given as

$$y = - T * (dy/dt) + G * x$$

in which x is the input forcing, a function of time; y is the response; dy/dt, its derivative; and T and G are two parameters characterizing the filter. T is the time constant, the time it would take the value of y to decay to 37% of its initial value in the absence of any input. G is the "static gain" or the ratio of output to input when the product of time constant and rate of change of y can be ignored. When their product is significant, as at high frequencies or for large time constants, the ratio of y to x is reduced from its maximum value of G. In the simulations of this chapter G is assumed to be 1, but this could be an additional option selected by the user of the program.

One method of digital solution is to use the Euler integration approximation used in many of the simulations of the previous chapters. Using such a method the integration interval must be small relative to the time constant of the process and thus may require storage and handling of a large number of digitized samples of the input waveform. This chapter uses an alternative method which is not subject to this restraint and in which the error is limited only by the precision of the arithmetic operations, not by the intervals between successive samples of the input forcing function, x. The reader is referred to the references at the end of this chapter for a rigorous treatment of the subject of digital filters but the discussion here is limited to developing an intuitive view of what the method involves.

AUTOREGRESSIVE DIFFERENCE EQUATION

The differential equation given above considers x and y as continous functions of time, such as x(t) and y(t), respectively. In digital simulations these continuous functions are sampled or computed at finite time increments, e.g. the DT=0.01 seconds used in the figures. The digitized functions can be stored and referenced in arrays, such as X(I) and Y(I), where the index I indicates the number of time increments DT, i.e., t=I*DT. It is possible to set up a "difference equation" relating Y(I) and X(I) which will be exactly equivalent to the differential equation for the continous variables x(t) and y(t). Knowing the parameters of the first-order process (T and G) and the successive values of X(I), which consists of samples of

x(t), it is possible to compute the solution Y(I), corresponding
to the exact solution of y(t) at the increments DT.    Although
there  are limitations upon the range of DT, it is not necessary
to make its value diminishingly small for  overall  accuracy  of
the filter.

        The first-order "autoregressive difference equation"  in
BASIC  format  equivalent  to  the above continuous differential
equation is

        Y(I) = ALPHA * Y(I-1) + G * (1 - ALPHA) * X(I).

This  indicates  that  each  new  output  Y(I)  is  computed  by
multiplying  the previous output, Y(I-1), by a coefficient ALPHA
and adding the current  input  sample  X(I)  multiplied  by  two
terms.    G is the static gain, defined before, and which we are
setting to unity.  The coefficient ALPHA depends upon  both  the
time  constant  T  of the process, and the sampling increment DT
according to the relation

        ALPHA = EXP(-DT/T).

This coefficient tells how much of the value  of  a  first-order
decay of y(t) will remain after an increment of time equal to DT
has transpired.

        Consider the special case for the difference equation in
which there is no input X(I) so that successive values of  Y(I)
are  always  the fraction ALPHA of the immediately previous one,
Y(I-1).  This decaying process is first  order,  with  the  rate
directly  proportional  to  what  remains.    Furthermore,  this
recursively computed solution is exact since ALPHA is based upon
the  time  constant  T  and  the  sampling  increment  DT.   The
situation is  analogous  to  calculating  radioactive  decay  at
multiples of the half-life in which the computation increment is
very large relative to the time constant of the decay.

        In  the  total difference equation the amount of Y(I) is
determined not only by what is left of the  previous  value  but
also by how much X(I) is added to it.  The terms G and (1-ALPHA)
are concerned with the units of X(I) and Y(I) and set  the  gain
of the process.  In the static case, in which successive samples
of X(I) and Y(I) do not change, the decay of  Y(I)  due  to  the
factor  ALPHA  is  compensated  by the multiplication of X(I) by
(1-ALPHA) a factor greater than one.

        Thus  the  steps  in using the autoregressive difference
equation for digital filtering of  stored  samples  consists  of
setting  the  factor  ALPHA  for  the  given  time  constant and
sampling interval and starting the iteration with  Y(I)  as  the
initial  value  of  the solution.  The reader is invited to test
this  by  comparing  analytical  solutions  of  the  differential

equation for known forcing functions with tabular printouts of
the solution of the difference equation using a program written
in BASIC.

As an illustration, Table 11.1 reproduces part of the
BASIC listing at the end of the chapter in which the input is a
sine function at a frequency HZ and for which 251 output values
are plotted using I as an index. Line 5220 establishes the
coefficient ALPHA from the time constant T and the computation
increment DT. It also sets the initial value of Y to zero. The
FOR-NEXT loop goes through 251 steps updating Y by multiplying
the previous value by ALPHA and adding in (1-ALPHA) times the
sinusodial forcing function. The value 75 scales the function
for plotting purposes and line 5260 plots it for values of the
abscissa from 25 to 275.

---

Table 11.1

Autoregressive difference equation solution and
plotting for a sinusoidal forcing at a frequency HZ
for which there are 100 steps to one complete cyle.
Only the first two letters in the label ALPHA are
recognized by the BASIC language used.

```
5220 ALPHA=EXP(-DT/T):  Y=0
5240 FOR I= 0 TO 250
5250    Y=Y*AL + (1-AL) * 75 * SIN(2*PI*HZ*I/100)
5260    HPLOT 25 +I, 75-Y
5265 NEXT I
```

---

A later section describes the equivalent operations in
which the input functions are stored pressure and ECG values.
The major point to be emphasized is that digitized signals can
be "low-pass filtered" by a single-step operation in which a new
output is obtained from the sum of the previous output and the
present input, each weighted according to the time constant of
the filter and the sampling increment of the input data.

RESTORING DISTORTED WAVEFORMS

Frequently digital computation can correct the
distortion introduced by a measurement process. This is
particularly easy to do if the data samples are already
digitized and if the compensation is to overcome errors due to a

linear first-order filter of known time constant. This correction process is sometimes called "inverse filtering" since it involves applying a mathematical operation which is the inverse of that which models the instrument which made the distorted measurements. Since the filtering can be simulated by a convolution process the inverse operation is also called "deconvolution".

In the simplest case, if the measured output is G times the input the correction consists of multiplication by 1/G. If the waveform is distorted by low-pass filtering it can be restored by "high-pass" filtering by applying a difference equation to be given below. There are limitations to the extent of recovery, of course, but slight modifications of the simulations in this chapter demonstrate the remarkable capabilities of inverse filtering. The application should become popular as digital technqiues become commonplace in audio and instrumentation recording.

Let us consider a digital method for recovering the sequence X(I) from the sequence Y(I) produced by the first-order difference equation given above. The samples of the restored waveform are called W(I) to distinguish them from the original true values of the quantity X(I). The difference equation which performs the inverse filtering is

    W(I) = Y(I)/(1-ALPHA) - Y(I-1)*ALPHA/(1-ALPHA).

As before, ALPHA is the decay of Y(I) during the interval DT. If the static gain is other than unity the factor G is included in the denominator of each of the terms on the right side of the equation. Thus the restoration consists of the difference between successive values of the distorted waveform each weighted according to the time constant of the filter and the sampling interval, an operation which can be performed in one line of a computer program.

The author has demonstrated this inverse filtering as an extension of the filtering simulations illustrated earlier in this chapter. At the resolution of the microcomputer display the restored waveform is indistinguishable from the original input, even when the filters have time constants as long as four seconds such that the waveform is almost a straight line. Reproduction of these waveforms appears the same as in the figures given earlier except for the reversed roles of inputs and outputs. It is more helpful to consider a simple numerical exercise. Suppose that an input sequence of data samples is filtered by the following difference equation

        Y(I)      =    0.96 * Y(I-1)   +    0.04 * X(I)
        distorted                                   original

The corresponding difference equation for the inverse filter, designed by using ALPHA=0.96 as for T=4 and DT=.01, is

$$
\begin{array}{lll}
W(I) & = & (1/.04) * Y(I) & - & (.96/.04) * Y(I-1) \\
W(I) & = & 25 * Y(I) & - & 24 * Y(I-1) \\
\text{restored} & & \text{distorted} & &
\end{array}
$$

Table 11.2 gives several successive values of the distorted variable Y(I) and the computed restoration W(I) when the input forcing X(I) is a step from 0 to 1 between I=0 and I=1. The computed Y(I) is an exponential rise toward a steady-state value of 1, the response characteristic of a low-pass filter subjected to a step input. The accuracy of the restored waveform is determined by the precision of the individual numerical operations involved.

---

Table 11.2

Digital computation of the response of a first-order process to a step change in input forcing by use of a difference equation. The original input can be recovered by applying a second difference equation which acts as an inverse filter.

| I<br>Index | X(I)<br>Input | Y(I)<br>Distorted | W(I)<br>Restored |
|---|---|---|---|
| 0 | 0 | 0 | 0 |
| 1 | 1 | .04 + 0   = .04 | 1.0 -  0 = 1 |
| 2 | 1 | .04 +.0384 = .0784 | 1.96- .96 = 1 |
| 3 | 1 | .04 +.0753 = .1153 | 2.88-1.88 = 1 |
| 4 | 1 | .04 +.1107 = .1507 | 3.77-2.77 = 1 |
| . | . | . | . |
| . | . | . | . |
| 999 | 1 | .04 +.96  = 1 | 25 -24  = 1 |
| 1000 | 1 | .04 +.96  = 1 | 25 -24  = 1 |

> THE BASIC PROGRAM

     This section describes the main features of a program written in BASIC which performs the simulations given in this chapter. The purpose is to document the complete listing given in the following Chapter Appendix and to provide information about where the program would have to be modified for different microcomputers.

     Initiation of the program consists of setting the variables PI and DT. A title panel with instructions is displayed while the arterial pressure and ECG data samples are being read from DATA statements into arrays P(I) and ECG(I) by the subroutine at line 8000 in the appendix. These data consist of 250 samples of each waveform at time increments of 0.01 seconds. The screen then displays the text shown in Figure 11.1A and asks for the input waveform option. When this is answered the program branches to routines at lines 5000, 6000, or 7000 depending upon the waveform selected.

     Lines 5000-5300 are involved with generating and displaying the sinusoidal input and computed response. These are scaled so that the input waveform has a peak value of 75 units above and below an ordinate of 75 as the zero line. The time increments are considered as 0.01 seconds so that the 250 displayed values constitute a total time span of 2.5 seconds. At a frequency of 1 Hz there are 100 points on the sine wave so that the waveform appears almost continuous as in Figure 11.1B. As the frequency increases above 5 Hz, where the period is less than 0.2 sec. with fewer than 20 points per cycle, the sinusoidal nature of the curves is obscured. The recursive computation of the response, in line 5250, was discussed in connection with Table 11.1 previously. The sinusoidal input values are computed at the time the output is computed which makes this simulation execute a bit slower than if they were stored in array as is done with the other waveforms.

     The routine at line 6000 is used for the arterial pressure waveform as an input to the filter. The axes and labels are drawn in the graphic mode and the 250 pressure values read from the data array. Table 11.3 reproduces the portion of the listing which computes the filtered pressure waveforms according to the selected time constant. Line 6190 sets the ALPHA coefficient appropriate for the value of T and DT. It also sets the initial value of output pressure, Y.

     The FOR-NEXT loop in lines 6200-6210 compute and plot 251 values of the output waveform using the difference equation. Each new value of Y is the sum of ALPHA times the previous Y plus the present pressure input P(I) times (1-ALPHA). This

value of Y is plotted above a baseline which is 150 lines  below
the  top  of  the  screen.  Note that the filtering is done in a
single BASIC statement.  The rest of the  program  is  concerned
with  plotting  axes  and asking for the filter parameters.  For
demonstrations  of  inverse  filtering  the   computed   output
responses are saved in an array from which the restored waveform
can be calculated as described above.

---

Table 11.3

BASIC  routine for computing first-order  response  with
time constant T at time  increments  DT  for  pressure
inputs stored in array P(I).  Each new value of output
Y is computed from the  previous  value  and  the  new
input pressure from the array.


6180 REM  -- PLOT FILTERED PRESSURE RECURSIVELY --
6190 ALPHA = EXP(-DT/T): INPUT Y
6200 FOR I=1 TO 250: Y = AL*Y + (1-AL)*P(I)
6210   HPLOT I+25, 150-Y
6215 NEXT I

---

     The routine at line 7000 plots the ECG input waveform on
the  top  half  of  the screen with a baseline which is 65 units
from the top of the screen.  Once the time constant is  selected
the computation is the same as for the pressure except the input
comes from the array ECG(I).  The baseline for  the  output  is
display  is  140  units  down  on the screen, separating the two
waveforms for clarity.  There are no axes  or  scales  displayed
with  the ECG since these seem to distract from the point of the
display.

REFERENCES

Agarwal, P., and R. Priemer: Microprocessor-based digital signal processing system. Comput. Biol. Med. 9:87-95 (1979).

Box, G. E. P., and G. M. Jenkins: Time Series Analysis forecasting and control. San Francisco: Holden-Day (1970).

Jenkins, G. M., and D. G. Watts: Spectral Analysis and Its Applications. San Francisco: Holden-Day (1969).

Lynn, P. A.: Recursive digital filters for biological signals. Med. & Biol. Engng. 9:37-43 (1971).

Murphy, D., and A. A. Dickie: Practical considerations in the design of fast lowpass recursive digital filters for biomedical applications. Med. & Biol. Engr. & Computing, 17:382-386 (1979).

Otnes, R. K., and L. Enochson: Digital Time Series Analysis. New York: John Wiley & Sons (1972).

Taylor, T. P., and P. W. Macfarlane: Digital filtering of the ECG. Med. & Biol. Engng. 12:493-503 (1974).

CHAPTER APPENDIX

The following pages contain a listing of the Applesoft BASIC routines which produce the simulations presented in this chapter. Lines 90 and 100 call in a machine-language routine and a character table used in the subroutine at line 5500 to place text on the high-resolution graphic displays.

```
10   REM    --  RECURSIVE DIGITAL FILTER  --
20   REM    FIRST-ORDER FILTERING OF
25   REM     SINE, PRESSURE, ECG WAVEFORMS
30   REM    APPLESOFT ON ROM AND 48K MEMORY
40 :
50 :
60   PRINT D$;"BLOAD CHARACTER TABLE $6800"
70 : REM    LOAD HI-RES ASCII CHARACTERS FROM DISK BELOW LOWMEM
80  D$ =  CHR$ (4)
90   PRINT D$;"BLOAD CHARACTER TABLE $6800"
100   PRINT D$;"BLOAD HI-RES CHARACTER GEN $6000"
110 :
120 :
130 :
1000   REM    -- INITIALIZATION --
1010   LOMEM: 32000: CLEAR : DIM P(250),ECG(250)
1020 PI = 3.1415926:DT = 0.01: TEXT : HOME
1030   GOSUB 4000: REM   TITLE,INSTRUCT. WHILE FILLING ARRAYS
1040   GOSUB 8000: REM   MOVE ECG,A.P. DATA INTO ARRAYS
1050 :
1060 :
1070 :
2000   REM    -- PICK INPUT OPTION --
2010   TEXT : HOME
2020   VTAB 4: HTAB 10: PRINT "RECURSIVE FILTERING"
2030   VTAB 7: HTAB 1: PRINT "INPUT TO THE FILTER:"
2040   VTAB 9: HTAB 5: PRINT "1) SINE WAVE"
2050   VTAB 11: HTAB 5: PRINT "2) ARTERIAL PRESSURE WAVEFORM"
2060   VTAB 13: HTAB 5: PRINT "3) ECG TRACING"
2070   VTAB 17: HTAB 20: INPUT "WHICH ? ";Z
2080   ON Z GOTO 5000,6000,7000
2090   GOTO 2000
2100 :
2110 :
2120 :
4000   REM    --- TITLE AND INSTRUCTIONS ---
4010   VTAB 5: HTAB 5: PRINT "DEMONSTRATION OF"
4020   HTAB 10: VTAB 8: PRINT "RECURSIVE FILTERING OF"
4030   HTAB 15: VTAB 11: PRINT "CARDIOVASCULAR WAVEFORMS"
4040   VTAB 18: PRINT "TO RESTART THE EXERCISE:"
4050   PRINT : PRINT "  PRESS RETURN WITHOUT ENTERING"
4060   PRINT : PRINT "    VALUE FOR TIME CONSTANT"
4070   RETURN
4080 :
4090 :
```

```
5000    REM    -- SINE WAVE FORCING --
5010    HTAB 1: VTAB 21
5015    PRINT "SELECT FREQUENCY OF SINUSOIDAL INPUT"
5020    HTAB 1: VTAB 23: PRINT "FREQUENCY (0-5 HZ) = ";
5030    HTAB 30: VTAB 23: PRINT "HZ";
5040    HTAB 24: VTAB 23: INPUT HZ
5050    HTAB 30: VTAB 23: PRINT "HZ";
5055    :
5060    REM  PLOT AXES AND LABELS
5070    HGR : HPLOT 25,75 TO 275,75
5080    FOR XX = 25 TO 275 STEP 25: HPLOT XX,73 TO XX,77: NEXT XX
5090    HPLOT 23,0 TO 23,150
5100    FOR YY = 0 TO 150 STEP 37.5: HPLOT 21,YY TO 22,YY: NEXT YY
5110    HTAB 2: VTAB 10:A$ = "0": GOSUB 5500
5120    HTAB 19: VTAB 9:A$ = "1": GOSUB 5500
5130    HTAB 33: VTAB 9:A$ = "2   SEC": GOSUB 5500
5135    :
5140    REM     PLOT SINUSODIAL INPUT WAVEFORM
5150    FOR I = 0 TO 250
5160    HPLOT 25 + I,075 - 075 *  SIN (2 * PI * HZ * I / 100)
5170    NEXT I
5180    HTAB 1: VTAB 24
5185    :
5190    INPUT "FILTER TIME CONSTANT = ? ";T$
5200    HTAB 30: VTAB 23: PRINT "SEC."
5210    IF T$ = "" THEN   GOTO 2000
5220    T =   VAL (T$):ALPHA =  EXP ( - DT / T):Y = 0
5225    :
5230    REM     PLOT OUTPUT RECURSIVELY
5240    FOR I = 0 TO 250
5250    Y = Y * AL + (1 - AL) * 75 *  SIN (2 * PI * HZ * I / 100)
5260    HPLOT 25 + I,75 - Y: NEXT I
5270    GOTO 5190
5280    :
5290    :
5300    :
5310    :
5320    :
5500    REM    -- PRINT A$ AS HI-RES CHAR --
5510    REM       TRANSFERS PRINT OPERATION TO
5515    REM          SUBROUTINE AT PAGE 96 ($6000)
5520 P1 =   PEEK (54):P2 =   PEEK (55)
5530    PR# 0: POKE 54,0: POKE 55,96
5540    PRINT A$;
5550    POKE 54,P1: POKE 55,P2: POKE   - 16301,0
5560    RETURN
5570    :
5580    :
5590    :
```

```
6000   REM    -- DISPLAY PRESSURE TRACING --
6010   HGR : VTAB 21: HTAB 4: PRINT "0";
6020   VTAB 21: HTAB 33: PRINT "2 SEC.";
6030   VTAB 21: HTAB 19: PRINT "1";
6040   HPLOT 25,150 TO 275,150: FOR XX = 25 TO 275 STEP 50
6050   HPLOT XX,151 TO XX,154: NEXT XX
6060   HPLOT 25,0 TO 25,150
6070   FOR YY = 0 TO 150 STEP 25: HPLOT 23,YY TO 24,YY: NEXT YY
6080   HTAB 1: VTAB 7:A$ = "100": GOSUB 5500
6090   HTAB 1: VTAB 19:A$ = "0": GOSUB 5500
6100   HTAB 15: VTAB 1:A$ = "ARTERIAL PRESSURE": GOSUB 5500
6110   FOR I = 1 TO 250: HPLOT I + 25,150 - P(I): NEXT I
6115 :
6120   REM    SELECT FILTER PARAMETERS
6130   POKE 34,22: HTAB 1: VTAB 24: INPUT "INIT.PRESS.=";Y$
6140   IF Y$ = "" THEN  GOTO 2000
6150   POKE 33,20: POKE 32,17: HOME
6160   INPUT "TIME CONSTANT=?";T$
6170 T =  VAL (T$): IF T$ = "" THEN  GOTO 2000
6175 :
6180   REM    PLOT FILTERED PRESSURE RECURSIVELY
6190 ALPHA =  EXP ( - DT / T):Y =  VAL (Y$)
6200   FOR I = 1 TO 250:Y = AL * Y + (1 - AL) * P(I)
6210   HPLOT I + 25,150 - Y: NEXT I
6220   GOTO 6160
6230 :
6240 :
6250 :
7000   REM   -- DISPLAY ECG --
7010   HGR : HTAB 15: VTAB 1:A$ = "FILTER INPUT:": GOSUB 5500
7020   FOR I = 1 TO 250: HPLOT I + 25,65 - 0.5 * ECG(I): NEXT I
7025 :
7030   REM    PICK FILTER PARAMETERS
7040   HTAB 15: VTAB 12:A$ = "FILTER OUTPUT:": GOSUB 5500
7050   HTAB 1: VTAB 22:
7060   INPUT "TIME CONSTANT (SECONDS) = ? ";T$
7070   IF T$ = "" THEN  GOTO 2000
7075 :
7080   REM    PLOT FILTERED ECG RECURSIVELY
7090 T =  VAL (T$):ALPHA =  EXP ( - DT / T):Y = 0
7100   FOR I = 1 TO 250:Y = Y * AL + (1 - AL) * ECG(I)
7110   HPLOT I + 25,140 - 0.5 * Y: NEXT I
7120   GOTO 7060
7130 :
7140 :
7150 :
7160 :
8000   REM    -- MOVE DATA INTO ARRAY --
8010   RESTORE : FOR I = 1 TO 250: READ P(I): NEXT I
8020   FOR I = 1 TO 250: READ EC(I): NEXT I: RETURN
8030 :
```

```
8040  REM    ----ARTERIAL PRESSURE AT DT=0.01 SEC----
8050  DATA   081,082,083,084,085,087,089,091,093,095
8060  DATA   099,101,104,105,107,109,110,112,115,117
8070  DATA   118,119,120,121,121,119,117,115,115,117
8080  DATA   118,117,116,115,114,113,112,112,111,110
8090  DATA   109,107,106,105,104,101,099,097,096,094
8100  DATA   093,092,091,090,090,088,087,087,086,085
8110  DATA   085,084,084,083,083,083,083,083,082,082
8120  DATA   082,082,082,081,081,081,081,080,080,080
8130  DATA   080,081,082,083,084,085,087,089,091,093
8140  DATA   095,099,101,104,105,107,109,110,112,115
8150  DATA   117,118,119,120,121,121,119,117,115,115
8160  DATA   117,118,117,116,115,114,113,112,112,111
8170  DATA   110,109,107,106,105,104,101,099,097,096
8180  DATA   094,093,092,091,090,090,088,087,087,086
8190  DATA   085,085,084,084,083,083,083,083,083,082
8200  DATA   082,082,082,082,081,081,081,081,080,080
8210  DATA   080,081,082,083,084,085,087,089,091,093
8220  DATA   095,099,101,104,105,107,109,110,112,115
8230  DATA   117,118,119,120,121,121,119,117,115,115
8240  DATA   117,118,117,116,115,114,113,112,112,111
8250  DATA   110,109,107,106,105,104,101,099,097,096
8260  DATA   094,093,092,091,090,090,088,087,087,086
8270  DATA   085,085,084,084,083,083,083,083,083,082
8280  DATA   082,082,082,082,081,081,081,081,080,080
8290  DATA   080,080,081,081,082,083,083,083,084,084
8310  REM    -----ECG DATA AT DT=0.01 SEC.-----
8320  DATA   003,007,009,010,010,011,010,010,009,008
8330  DATA   007,006,004,002,002,001,030,050,073,092
8340  DATA   056,005,-20,-10,-05,000,002,002,003,003
8350  DATA   004,005,007,010,015,018,018,018,017,015
8360  DATA   014,012,010,009,008,006,004,003,001,001
8370  DATA   -01,-02,-03,-03,-02,-02,-02,-01,-01,-01
8380  DATA   000,000,000,000,001,001,001,001,002,002
8390  DATA   002,001,002,001,001,000,000,-01,-01,000
8400  DATA   001,005,007,009,010,010,011,010,010,009
8410  DATA   008,007,006,004,002,002,001,030,050,073
8420  DATA   092,056,005,-20,-10,-05,000,001,002,003
8430  DATA   003,004,005,007,010,015,018,018,018,017
8440  DATA   015,014,012,010,009,008,006,004,003,001
8450  DATA   001,-01,-02,-03,-03,-02,-02,-02,-01,-01
8460  DATA   -01,000,000,000,000,001,001,001,001,002
8470  DATA   002,002,001,002,001,001,000,000,-01,-01
8480  DATA   000,001,005,007,009,010,010,011,010,010
8490  DATA   009,008,007,006,004,002,002,001,030,050
8500  DATA   073,092,056,005,-20,-10,-05,000,001,002
8510  DATA   003,003,004,005,007,010,015,018,018,018
8520  DATA   017,015,014,012,010,009,008,006,004,003
8530  DATA   001,001,-01,-02,-03,-03,-02,-02,-02,-01
8540  DATA   -01,-01,000,000,000,000,001,001,001,001
8550  DATA   002,002,002,001,002,001,001,000,000,-01
8560  DATA   -01,000,001,005,007,009,010,010,010,011
```

Chapter 12


AXON ACTION POTENTIALS


The programs described in this chapter serve two
purposes. First, they permit the use of microcomputers
containing graphic display features to simulate the classical
teaching exercise about action potentials in nerves excised from
frogs. The computer routine asks for the amplitude and duration
parameters for two electrical stimuli separated in time. The
model then solves for the membrane conductances to Na+ and to
K+, the major ionic currents, and the transmembrane potential
which would be expected as a consequence of the stimuli. The
stimulus amplitude and membrane potential are displayed as they
are computed to give plots similar to the analog oscilloscope
preparations using living tissue. This microcomputer simulation
is convenient for lecture demonstrations and provides an
opportunity for independent self-study of the properties of axon
excitation by students. The computer does not provide practice
in tissue dissection, but it does direct full attention to the
physiological properties without the problems encountered by
unskilled experimenters.

A second feature of the simulation is that it can
provide insight about the hypothesized mechanisms involved in
excitation in a way that is not practical with animal
preparations. For example, graphs of membrane conductances show
the difference in timing of the increases in Na+ and in K+
permeabilities and the way these do not respond to stimuli
during the refractory period. Tabular presentations of membrane

James E. Randall, Microcomputers and Physiological Simulation

currents illustrate that threshold is the condition in which Na+
entry into the axon exceeds K+ loss in a regenerative way.
Furthermore, if the computer program is written in BASIC this
coding of logical, iterative steps is a method of communicating
the dynamic essence of the excitation process.

The effectiveness of the simulation lies not in the
programming but in the durability of the classic work Hodgkin
and Huxley did upon the squid axon and published in a set of
four papers in 1952. The first three of these established
empirical relationships for the voltage- and time-dependence of
membrane conductance changes following a clamped step change in
membrane voltage. The fourth paper (Hodgkin and Huxley, 1952)
showed, through simulation, that the kinetics of the
conductances could account for conduction and excitation in
quantitative terms. These formulations, though modified in
detail, are still the standard textbook explanations for a wide
range of physiological properties, including threshold, temporal
summation, stimuli strength-duration relationship,
accommodation, refractoriness, anode-break excitation, and
firing freqeuncy as a function of stimulus amplitude. Their
original computations, taking hours to days, can be reproduced
within seconds on modern microcomputers making the simulations
realistic for teaching exercises.

The Hodgkin-Huxley equations (HH-Eq) have been fully
described, analyzed, tested, and computed over the years so the
attention of this chapter is focused upon how to implement them
in microcomputers. The tabular outputs which give successive
values of conductances, currents, and voltage following stimuli
can be run on almost any microcomputer having BASIC. The time
involved on successive iterations is significant but about
matches the time it takes to read and digest what is happening
on the screen. The graphic displays of variables require that
the computer have a degree of plotting resolution in order to be
effective. Also, computation speed is important and a numerical
processor chip (discussed in Chapter 4) is advisable so that a
variety of stimulus parameters can be tested in a reasonable
time.

The programs presented here are organized for
convenience of documentation not for execution speed. The
language used is Microsoft BASIC which is common in personal
microcomputers such as the TRS-80, Apple II, and those using
CP/M. A main routine is given which calls individual
subroutines dedicated to specialized tasks. This permits us to
talk about these individually and present alternative methods
for accomplishing them on the different computers and for
different teaching objectives. Special sections are devoted to
output displays and to computation methods involving the
compromise between speed and accuracy. At this point the
simulations are related to the properties of excitation by

illustrative  material from which self-teaching exercises can be
designed.

The use of a numerical processor chip to achieve graphic
simulations within a few seconds is technical but a separate
section is included giving the general principles to be followed
by those having assembly-language skills. It is only a matter
of time until the more convenient high-level languages are
designed around numerical processors in order to realize their
speed advantages. The reader is referred to the excellent
chapter by Dr. Peter Stewart (1973) which contains FORTRAN
listings of routines which he has used for teaching-simulations
through terminals accessing the large computers at Brown
University.

```
┌──────────────────────────┐
│   FORMULATION IN BASIC    │
└──────────────────────────┘
```

The  steps  in the teaching simulation consist of asking
for the stimuli parameters (amplitude, duration, and delay);
asking for the initial steady-state membrane potential and for a
step change in voltage, if desired; and then executing
successive iterations of computuations and displays of
variables.

The computation steps consist of determining the
membrane conductances as voltage- and time-dependent variables
described by nonlinear differential equations; using these
conductances and associated driving forces to establish the
membrane currents; and then adding these inward and outward
currents, along with the stimulus, if any, to establish the net
rate at which charged particles are crossing the membrane. The
membrane voltage is updated according to the net charge which is
transferred during a finite computation interval. Graphic and
tabular outputs of the computed variables of interest are
included within an iteration.

Table 12.1 lists the main computing routine which calls
subroutines to perform the special operations though this
modular organization may be inefficient for computational
purposes. This permits us to consider alternative methods of
performing the individual steps as required by the computer
being used and the teaching objectives.

Lines 100 to 700 determine the stimuli and set up the
initial values of variables. Lines 800 to 1500 call subroutines
which do the computation and display the output. The subroutine
called from line 100 supplies the queries asking for the
amplitudes and durations of the stimulating currents. In line
300 the computing increment used in the Euler integrations is
set to 1/25 msec, a compromise between accuracy and speed which

is satisfactory for teaching purposes. Alternative methods of performing the numerical integration and for picking the integration time interval are discussed in greater detail in a later section.

---

Table 12.1

An overview of the steps in the simulation of an action potential. The first section sets up the stimulus and the initial steady-state values. The iteration loop calculates the membrane conductances and currents which are considered to be constant through the time interval T to T+DT. The total current flowing during the time increment DT is used to compute a new membrane voltage. Then the process is repeated. Output may be either numerical tables or graphic plots.

```
100 REM   -- HODGKIN-HUXLEY MODEL FOR SQUID AXON --
200 GOSUB 2000        (Get stimulus parameters
300 T=0: DT=1/25      (Initialize time, increment
400 MV=-90            (Initial steady-state voltage
500 GOSUB 3000        (Set alpha's, beta's for volts
600 GOSUB 3200        (Set steady-state N, M, H
700 GOSUB 3500        (Set init. conduct, currents
799 :
800 REM    LOOPS BACK HERE AFTER EACH ITERATION <---
900 GOSUB 4000        (Display variables
1000 GOSUB 3000       (Set alpha, beta's for new V
1100 GOSUB 5000       (Update conductances
1200 GOSUB 5500       (Update currents
1300 GOSUB 5700       (Update voltage
1400 T=T+DT           (Increment time
1500 GOTO 900         (Repeat at new voltage ----->
1510 :
```

---

Line 400 sets the initial resting membrane potential to a value of -90 millivolts. In demonstrations of anode-break excitation this could start from a more negative value as chosen by the operator. The subroutine called in line 500 sets a number of first-order rate constants which vary only with membrane potential. The subroutine at line 3200, called in line 600, uses these rate constants to determine the steady-state values of three dimensionless variables associated with the temporal changes of membrane conductances to Na+ and to K+. These are used by the next subroutine to set up the initial membrane conductances and currents.

Table 12.2

Symbols and steady-state values of the variables  used
in the  simulations.   These follow the notation and
conventions of the  original  papers  by  Hodgkin  and
Huxley.


| SYMBOL | VARIABLE | STEADY-STATE VALUE |
|--------|----------|--------------------|
| SA(1) | Stim #1, amplitude | ??? µamp/sq cm |
| SD(1) | Stim #1, duration | ??? msec |
| SA(2) | Stim #2, amplitude | ??? µamp/sq cm |
| SD(2) | Stim #2, duration | ??? msec |
| DLY | Delay to #2 | ??? msec |
| | | |
| AN | Alpha-N, K+ off-on | 0.058 /msec |
| BN | Beta-N,  K+ on-off | 0.125 /msec |
| AM | Alpha-M, Na+ off-on | 0.224 /msec |
| BM | Beta-M,  Na+ on-off | 4.0   /msec |
| AH | Alpha-H  Na+ off-on | 0.07  /msec |
| BH | Beta-H   Na+ on-off | 0.047 /msec |
| | | |
| N | K+ activation | 0.318 |
| M | Na+ activation | 0.053 |
| H | Na+ inactivation | 0.596 |
| | | |
| GK | K+ conductance | 0.367  m.mho/sq cm |
| GNA | Na+ conductance | 0.010      " |
| | | |
| IK | K+ current | -4.40  µamp/sq cm |
| INA | Na+ current | 1.22      " |
| IL | Leakage current | 3.18      " |
| IT | Total current | 0.0      " |
| | | |
| | Membrane voltage | |
| MV | inside – outside | -90   mvolts |
| V | displace.from rest | 0   mvolts |

The first time through the iterative loop line 900 calls
the output display subroutine to show the baseline values of the
variables  of  interest.    Subsequent  times  around  the  loop  it
shows  the new values as  updated  by  the  remaining  subroutine
calls.   These perform to set the rate constants (line 1000), the
conductances  (line 1100),  the  currents  (line  1200),  and  the
voltage  (line  1300).   The final step is to increment the time
variable  by  the  integration  interval  DT  and then repeat the

iteration. Depending upon the output display format other branching logic may be needed. For instance, to graph several milliseconds onto the CRT it may be necessary to complete several computation loops between each call to the output display routine.

Several computations per displayed line may be necessary in tables of numerical output. This format may also require replacing the column labels as the computation lines scroll off the top of the CRT screen. In addition, it is possible to have within this loop statements that test the keyboard for commands to pause or to restart the simulation.

Table 12.2 lists the variables used in the simulations of this chapter along with their steady-state values. Though Microsoft BASIC uses only the first two letters of the symbols for variables, in many cases the third letter is included for clarity. For example, DLY for delay, INA for sodium current, and GNA for sodium conductance. Each of the variables in the table are defined within the context of their use in the computer routine.

A special notice should be taken of the conventions for voltage and current. Hodgkin and Huxley presented their empirical equations for conductance rate constants in terms of the membrane potential as displaced from resting value. According to their convention, which used the symbol V, depolarizations were negative while hyperpolarizations were positive. Modern microelectrode measurements use the convention of referring intracellular potentials to the extracellular sink as a reference. This variable is denoted by the symbol MV. Thus the subroutines carry statements which convert between these two conventions.

The author rather arbitrarily chose a resting membrane potential of -90 mv though values between -70 and -90 are often used in textbooks. The following discussions will use the convention of having positive currents for a net entry of positive ions acting to reduce the intracellular negativity. The term "inward current" will be used in the sense of having positive ions enter the axon.

INITIAL CONDITIONS

We shall now consider each of the subroutines called by the initialization routine given in lines 100-700 above. The subroutine starting in line 2000, called from line 200, simply asks for the stimulus parameters as identified in Table 12.2. The amplitudes, durations, and delay are meaningful values so there is no need to use normalized values as is done with the model in the previous chapter. The idea is to mimic the setting

of the dials on an electronic stimulator as used in a
neurophysiology laboratory. Default values of the variables
could be set to zero for the first run of an exercise but left
"as is" for subsequent runs to speed up entries when only one
parameter is to be changed. The subroutine would contain
statements such as

```
2000 REM    --  GET STIMULI PARAMETERS  --
2100 INPUT "Stimulus #1 amplitude =";SA(1)
2200 ...
2300 ...
2999 RETURN
```

In addition to acquiring parameters it is also important to test
for "out of limit" entries to avoid unrealistic responses for
the amplitude and time scales of the graphic displays.

There are teaching circumstances in which it would be
advantageous to start from a hyperpolarized condition, as in
demonstrating anode-break excitation. In this case the
subroutine at line 2000 could ask for the desired initial
membrane potential and then ask for the desired potential at the
start of the simulation. By using the resting membrane
potential as the default values for both queries by the computer
the student can quickly skip over these steps. The photograph
in Figure 12.1 shows the responses which have been entered to
test for axon excitability by applying two identical stimului
separate in time. In this case the student has skipped over the
opportunity to change the initial membrane potential from its
resting value of -90 mv.

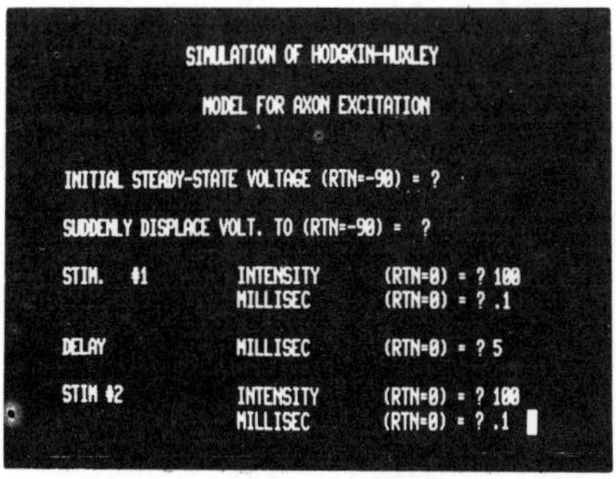

Fig. 12.1. CRT screen after
entering the amplitudes and
durations for two identical
stimuli separated by 5 msec.
This display could have 16
lines of 64 characters each.

Once the stimulus values have been set it is necessary to
intitialize certain variables according to the chosen initial
membrane potential. Subroutines called from lines 500 through
700 perform this, but it is most instructive to consider the
last of these first. Table 12.3 has the subroutine starting at
line 3500 which sets the initial steady-state membrane currents

according to the electrochemical driving potentials and
conductances for the major permeable ions.

The calculation of permeable ion currents follows
standard logic of a driving force factor and a conductance
factor. In line 3550 the driving force is denoted by (V-12)
where V is the voltage expressed as a displacement from resting
value. The number 12 is a measure of the concentration gradient
for K+ determined by the activity (concentration) ratio of this
ion across the membrane and the temperature according to the
Nernst equation. The flexiblity of the teaching exercise can be
increased by having the protocal ask for intracellular and
extracellular concentrations of each major ion. In the present
case, if the membrane is hyperpolarized to V=+12, there is no
net driving force upon the K+ ions.

```
                        Table 12.3

    The subroutine at line 3500 which sets membrane
    conductances and currents according to dimensionless
    variables determined by the initial membrane potential
    and by the electrochemical driving forces.


    3500 REM   -- INITIAL CONDUCTANCES AND CURRENTS --
    3510 :
    3520 GK  =   36 * N*N*N*N          (K+ conductance
    3530 GNA =  120 * M*M*M * H        (Na+      "
    3540 :
    3550 IK  =   GK * (V-12)           (K+   current
    3560 INA =  GNA * (V+115)          (Na+       "
    3570 IL  =  0.3 * (V+10.6)         (Leakage  "
    3580 :
    3590 IT  =  IK + INA + IL          (Total current
    3600 :
    3610 RETURN
```

Line 3560 calculates the Na+ current and indicates that
when the membrane is depolarized to V=-115 this ion will be in
electrochemical equilibrium. The leakage current, Cl- and other
ions, balances the currents of the other two ions so that the
total current IT adds to very nearly zero in line 3590. Note
that the conductance for this leakage current is a constant of
0.3 millimho/sq cm whereas those of the other two ions are
variables.

The contribution of Hodgkin's and Huxley's formulation
of the kinetics of membrane conductance changes appears in the

dimensionless factors N, for K+ in line 3520 and M and H for Na+
in line 3530. These workers found that when a squid axon's
membrane voltage was clamped at some new voltage the K+
permeability increased as though it involved the product of four
exponential expressions. They worked with a mathematical model
where N is a dimensionless variable falling within the range of
0 to 1 and which can be described by a first-order differential
equation. When a membrane is hyperpolarized the value of N
tends to be small and the K+ current is small; when depolarized,
N is large and K+ conductance can approach its maximum value of
36 millimho/sq cm, the value used in these formulations. During
voltage changes from one value to another N must be calculated
as a solution to a first-order differential equation.

Line 3530 indicates that Na+ conductance contains a
constant of 120, corresponding to the maximum possible
conductance, and the products of two other dimensionless
variables, M and H. The variable M, often called Na+
activation, is analogous to the variable N for K+ except that
its response is much faster and only three terms were involved
in the empirical fit to the squid axon data. The variable H,
Na+ inactivation, has a large value at resting potentials so
that with a stimulus Na+ current inititially is limited
primarily by the degree of turning on the Na+ activation
variable N. However, with increasing time after the stimulus
the inactivation factor H falls to values so low that it limits
Na+ current, an important component of the refractory period.
Note that it requires less computer time to calculate the
product of N four times than it does to use the more general
power function.

Now we can turn to the subroutines which establish the
steady-state values of the variables N, M, and H according to
the chosen value for the resting membrane potential. The finite
approximation to the defining differential equation describing
the kinetics of the variable N is given as

DN/DT = AN * (1-N) - BN * N

where DN is the change in N over the computing interval DT.
There is no known molecular basis for these kinetic models but
conceptually the variable N can be considered as the fraction of
some sites which are in the "ON" state and (1-N) is the fraction
of these sites in the "OFF" state. In order for K+ to traverse
a membrane channel it is necessary for four of these sites to be
simultaneously in the ON state, hence N*N*N*N corresponds to the
fraction of channels with these four sites being on. When N is
nearly one the full conductance of K+ can be realized.

In the above differential equation AN, normally called
alpha-n, gives the rate constant for conversion of OFF states to
ON states; BN, normally called beta-n, is the rate constant for

conversion of ON to OFF states. Similar differential equations
can be given for the rates of change of the variables M and H
using the rate constants AM and BM for the first and AH and BH
for the second.

In the steady state the rate of change of each of these
dimensionless variables is zero and the differential equation
can be solved to establish the variable from the correponding
rate constants. This is done in the subroutine at line 3200.

```
3200 REM  -- STEADY-STATE VARIABLES
3210 N = AN / (AN + BN)
3220 M = AM / (AM + BM)
3230 H = AH / (AH + BH)
3240 RETURN
```

According to the model the rate constants which
determine the kinetics of the dimensionless variables depend
upon membrane electric potential and not upon time. During the
course of an action potential the voltage is continually
changing, altering the individual rates at which the Na+ and K+
sites are changing to and from an ON state, and thus influencing
the membrane conductance in a complex way. It clearly requires
a computational aid to follow the multiplicity of dynamic
interacting factors. The durability of this model is a crowning
example of what simulation can do to illuminate the behavior of
complex biological systems. The model is empirical, however,
and has not identified the molecular mechanisms responsible for
the permeability changes it describes.

Table 12.4 gives the subroutine which calculates the
rate constants which correspond to the current membrane voltage.
Upon entering the subroutine at line 3000 the voltage
information is contained in the variable MV. Line 3020 offsets
this to the value V corresponding to a displacement from rest
potential. Note that in lines 3100 and 3110 there are
possibilities of a division by zero if the value of V equals -10
or -25. Therefore lines 3030 and 3040 test for these conditions
and provide slight offsets when the values do occur. This
appears to have no significant influence upon the solutions
within the limits of accuracy required for teaching purposes.

In considering the influence of changes of V upon these
rate constants it can be seen that for depolarizations (V<0) AM
tends to increase and BM to decrease, the two combining to
increase the variable M and thus enhance Na+ entry. However,
depolarization also decreases AH and increases BH, favoring
conversion of ON sites to OFF ones and the fall in the variable
H which describes Na+ inactivation. The rate constants of AH
and BH are about 0.1 times those of AM and BM which gives the
difference in timing of the activation and inactivation

processes hypothesized to be involved in the permeability changes of Na+ in excitable membranes.

---

Table 12.4

This subroutine calculates the rate constants in the first-order differential equations which fit the kinetics of the dimensionless parameters contained in the expressions for Na+ and K+ conductances. The rate constants are considered to respond to voltage instantaneously.

```
3000 REM  -- CALCULATE RATE CONSTANTS FOR VOLTAGE --
3010 :
3020 V = - MV - 90                      (V=0 at rest
3030 IF V+25 = 0 THEN V=-25.1           (Avoid 1/0
3040 IF V+10 = 0 THEN V=-10.1
3050 :
3060 BN = 0.125*EXP(V/80)               (Beta-N
3070 BM = 4*EXP(V/18)                    (Beta-M
3080 BH = 1/(EXP((V+30)/10)+1)           (Beta-H
3090 :
3100 AN = 0.01*(V+10)/(EXP((V+10)/10)-1) (Alpha-N
3110 AM = 0.1*(V+25)/(EXP((V+25)/10)-1)  (Alpha-M
3120 AH = 0.07*EXP(V/20)                 (Alpha-H
3130 :
3140 RETURN
3150 :
```

---

THE ITERATION LOOP

    With the stimulus parameters and steady-state values of variables established we are now ready to describe the iteration loop as listed in lines 900-1500 in Table 12.1. We have mentioned the kinetic rate constants and dimensionless variables which determine the conductance to Na+ and to K+ in the previous section. The main new factor to consider is the way that the values of N, M, and H are updated upon each iteration. For clarity we shall limit ourselves to Euler integration to update these variables upon each iteration using the rate constants appropriate for the present membrane voltage. A later section discusses alternative computational methods. Also we treat the output displays as a separate topic since they will vary according to the format desired and the hardware being used.

Line 900 calls whatever output display is given in a subroutine at line 4000. The specific point to be made here is that upon the first iteration this will display the steady-state values of variables as computed in lines 200-700. This serves the useful purpose of establishing base-line conditions before the stimulus is actually applied. The second time around the loop will report the results at the end of DT seconds and will include any stimulating current which is acting during the interval.

---

Table 12.5

Calculating new membrane conductances based upon rectangular integration approximations to the changes in the dimensionless parameters.

```
5000 REM   -- UPDATE CONDUCTANCES --
5010 :
5020 DN = (AN * (1-N) - BN * N) * DT     (Change in N
5030 DM = (AM * (1-M) - BM * M) * DT     (    "    in M
5040 DH = (AH * (1-H) - BH * H) * DT     (    "    in H
5050 :
5060 N = N + DN                          (New N
5070 M = M + DM                          (New M
5080 H = H + DH                          (New H
5090 :
5100 GK  =  36 * N*N*N*N
5110 GNA = 120 * M*M*M * H
5120 :
5130 RETURN
```

---

We have previously discussed the subroutine at line 3000 and since the rate constants are voltage-dependent and not time-dependent they will take on values determined by the value of V during the iteration. The new procedure involves updating the Na+ and K+ conductances by changing the variables N, M, and H according to their first-order differential equations. The computations are based upon the approximation of using a constant rate of change over the integration increment DT. Table 12.5 contains the BASIC statements. Line 5020 calculates the change DN in the K+ activation factor and line 5060 replaces the old N with the new one to be used for this iteration. The other lines do a similar modification upon the variables M and H. Before leaving the subroutine the old values of the conductances are replaced with the new ones in lines 5100 and 5110.

```
                        Table 12.6

Computation of currents during the time interval T  to
T+DT including stimulating current, if any.

5500 REM  -- CALCULATE NEW CURRENTS --
5520 IK  = GK  * (V-12)               (K+    Current
5530 INA = GNA * (V+115)              (Na+      "
5540 IL  = 0.3 * (V+10.6)             (Leakage "
5550 IT  =  IK + INA + IL             (Total    "
5560 :
5570 REM    IS THERE A STIMULUS TO ADD IN?
5580 IF T < SD(1) THEN IT = IT + SA(1)    (#1?
5590 IF T => (DLY + SD(2)) THEN RETURN    (#2?
5600 IF T => DLY THEN IT = IT + SA(2)     (#2
5610 :
5620 RETURN
```

The subroutine at line 5500 given in Table 12.6 calculates the currents as explained before but now must decide whether the stimulus current is to be included during the time interval, T to T+DT, being considered. If T is still during the interval of the first stimulus its value is added into the total membrane current in line 5580. If T has passed the end of the second stimulus, line 5590 causes an exit from the subroutine without any stimulus. If T is during the interval of the second stimulus which started some delay time after the start of the first one, line 5600 will add in its value.

When the total current IT is assumed to be constant during the integration increment DT, the product of these two terms indicates the total charge transferred across 1 sq cm of the axon wall. Since it is customary to use a membrane capacitance value of 1 microfarad/sq cm the calculation of the membrane voltage change DV during the interval DT does not involve numerical conversion but only units. The subroutine at line 5700 does this, taking into account that positive currents are depolarizing, and that the variable V becomes less than zero during depolarization.

```
5700 REM  -- NEW MEMBRANE VOLTAGE --
5710 DV =  IT * DT              (Cap = 1 μfd/sq cm
5720  V =   V - DV              (Displaced from rest
5730 MV = - V - 90              (Inside - outside
5740 RETURN
```

Line 5730 keeps the variable MV in the familiar frame of reference used today.

```
┌─────────────────────┐
│  OUTPUT DISPLAYS    │
└─────────────────────┘
```

The two kinds of CRT displays of computed variables to be discussed are numerical values in tabular form which scroll up on the screen at selected time increments and graphic displays which appear similar to analog oscilloscope tracings measured in the laboratory. The tabular values have the advantage of carrying several significant digits (as many as nine in Applesoft) which are helpful in comparing the relative values of Na+ and K+ currents for near-threshold stimuli. Also the time spent upon each iteration is less noticeable because the operator must concentrate upon the information being presented before it scrolls off the top of the screen. But, because only a few lines of output can be observed on the screen at one time it is easy to miss the overall pattern that a graph reveals. More information can be retained by a hard-copy printer but there are disadvantages associated with these mechanical devices. The best compromise appears to be to use tabular displays for a few first illustrative exercises to get across the large magnitudes of the currents during excitation compared to those at rest. Then, the bulk of the exercises resort to graphic displays which, out of necessity, have to be normalized to some scale to fit the screen.

TABULAR DISPLAYS

Considerations regarding displays of scrolling tables of computed variables evolve around the number of characters per line for the CRT, the particular variables of interest which can best reveal the property of excitation being demonstrated, and a time increment for the displays which catches the significant changes but still keeps the students' attention. CRT displays of 40 characters per line do not handle as many variables on a line but generally carry more lines giving a view through a wider window in time. In a previous chapter we mentioned the fact that Applesoft BASIC does not have a PRINT USING command, necessitating special tricks to keep the column aligned with a given number of digits. It should be recalled that the Apple II does have a special feature of fixing the scrolling window in any arbitrary area on the screen so that the column headings can remain in fixed position at the top of the screen.

The factors involved in the choice of the computing increment DT are discussed in the next section but in practice these prove to offer too fine a time resolution to be practical for line-by-line output. For example, at an increment of DT=1/25 msec over 25 lines are required to get to the peak of the action potential. Figures in later sections of this chapter show that

a printing increment of 0.2 msec is reasonable, each line  being
presented  after  either  5  computations with DT=0.04 or even 4
with DT=0.05 msec.  Of course  the  smaller  the  increment  the
greater the accuracy, but at a cost of computation speed.


TRS-80 GRAPHIC DISPLAYS

          There  are  many  factors  which  must  be considered in
designing a graphic  display  on  the  microcomputers  available
today.    These  are  illustrated for each of the three prototype
computers trying to point out the features  and  limitations  of
each.   Attention is focused upon the minimum requirements of the
subroutine at line 4000 which is called  at  the  first  of  the
iteration  loop  in  the  main  program  given  in  Table  12.1.
Generally  there  are  additional  statements  required  in  the
inititation  stages  which  clear  the screen, plot the axes and
tics, and put on any labels.  These are not dealt  with  in  any
detail.    In some of the CRT displays given in this chapter the
baselines  for  the  variables,  such  as  the  resting membrane
potential,  are plotted for several successive increments of the
abscissa before the simulation starts at  T=0.    The  computing
increment  DT  may  be  set  to  different values in each of the
following examples.


Fig.  12.2.   Illustrating the
graphic  capabilities  of  the
TRS-80  in  a demonstration of
the  refractory  period  where
the    second    stimulus   is
ineffective.  This  resolution
is  usable  within  limits and
the computer is  very  popular
because  of  its  initial  low
cost.

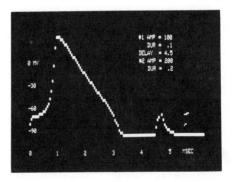

          The first one, the TRS-80, is limited to a resolution of
48 vertical by 128 horizontal positions which gives coarse  axes
lines  and  abrupt  discontinuities  in  the  curves  along with
limited time resolution.  Figure 12.2 is  an  action  potential
photographed  from  the  face of a video monitor attached to the
TRS-80 showing  the  computed  membrane  voltage  following  two
stimuli  separated  in time.  The vertical resolution is 10/3 mv
and the  temporal  resolution  is  0.05  msec,  the  computation
increment used.    In  this example the subroutine at line 2000
cleared the screen with a CLS command and  then  asked  for  and
displayed the numerical values of the stimulus parameters in the
upper right corner.

The plotting subroutine at line 4000 is very simple, consisting of only two lines.

```
4000 REM  -- TRS-80  PLOTTING ROUTINE --
4010 SET (INT(T/DT),35-INT((90+MV)/3))
4020 IF T >  6.25 THEN GOTO 4020
4030 RETURN
```

This uses the BASIC Level II command, not on all microcomputers, SET(X,Y) where X and Y are coordinates on a grid having the origin at the upper left corner. As T increases for each increment of DT (0.05 in this example) the x-coordinate is moved across the screen. At a resting potential of -90 mv the y-coordinate is 35 steps down on the screen. Line 4020 puts the program in a "software halt" after 6.25 msec. The display of much longer time spans requires more than one computation per display, increasing the computation time and decreasing the display resolution proportionately. These two factors make this hardware configuration awkward for demonstration of such features of excitation as the full time course of the refractory period, accommodation, and repeated firing for fixed inward current.

The TRS-80 does have the feature, not available on many microcomputers, of convenient intermixing of alphanumeric upper case letters with the graphics. In the display of Figure 12.2 the stimulus parameters stay in place during the simulation reminding the student of the conditions which are evoking the developing action potential.


S-100 GRAPHIC DISPLAYS

Most S-100 based computer owners have to configure their own hardware arrangements to include a graphic interface. The following discussion applies to one of many possible configurations which can serve as an example. The graphics interface, whose features are described in Chapter 4, is the Matrox capable of plotting either 256 or 240 vertical positions by 256 horizontal. As presented this is addressed through four of the 8080 microprocessor I/O ports using these Microsoft CP/M BASIC I/O commands:

```
OUT 7,0               will clear the screen
OUT 5,X               will set the x-coordinate
OUT 6,Y               will set the y-coordinate
WAIT 4,1,1:OUT 4,1    will turn on a dot at X,Y
```

The four I/O ports, numbered 4-7 here, are determined by hardware patches. The origin for the coordinate system is in the upper left-hand corner for this display board also.

The subroutine which is to be put at location 4000 for plotting on a CRT connected to the Matrox video board contains the features of that given in Table 12.7. According to the scheme given the x-coordinate advances one step for each iteration in line 4020. Line 4030 scales the MV variable to a 1.5 mv resolution and plots it relative to a zero line 40 units down on the screen.

---

### Table 12.7

Subroutine to be called from main iteration loop to put computed variables onto a Matrox 256 x 240 point display. Each variable appears as a scaled deflection from a zero-value line. The stimulus amplitude ST is set depending upon the value of the time variable T.

```
4000 REM   -- MATROX PLOTS OF VARIABLES --
4010 :
4020 OUT 5,INT(T/DT)                (Set x-
4030 OUT 6,40 -(MV/1.5)             (Set y-
4040 WAIT 4,1,1:OUT 4,1             (Plot mv
4050 :
4060 OUT 6,238-(150*N*N*N*N)        (Normal. GK
4070 WAIT 4,1,1:OUT 4,1             (Plot it
4080 :
4090 OUT 7,238-(150*M*M*M*H)        (Normal. GNa
4100 WAIT 4,1,1:OUT 4,1             (Plot it
4110 :
4120 REM  PLOT STIMULUS, IF ANY
4130 ST=0
4140 IF T <SD(1) THEN ST=SA(1)      (Stim #1
4150 IF T=> DLY AND T <(DLY+SD(2))
       THEN ST=ST+SA(2)             (Stim #2
4160 OUT 6,160-(ST/5)               (Set Y
4170 WAIT 4,1,1:OUT 4,1             (Plot Stim
4180 :
4190 RETURN
```

---

In order to follow the relative time courses of the Na+ and K+ conductances these are normalized by taking the products of their respective dimensionless variables and also a scaling factor of 150. This is shown in line 4060 and 4090 where they are each plotted above a zero line at Y=238 near the bottom of the screen. The stimulus current could have been set to a separate variable back in another subroutine which included the total membrane current, but for clarity it is done here where it is used. Lines 4130 to 4150 set the variable ST depending upon

whether T falls within the time of a stimulus. ST is then scaled
down by a factor of 5 and plotted above a zero line at Y=160.

        Figure 12.3 shows the results of computing and  plotting
the  responses of two equal stimuli separated by a delay time of
5 msec.  Though there are no labels on these plots it is easy to
identify    the    stimulus    in    the    middle  tracing  and  the
corresponding  depolarization  responses  in  the  top  tracing.
After  the  first  stimulus there is a regenerative response but
not after the second.  The bottom tracings show the  rapid  rise
in  Na+  conductance  and  the slower, more sustained rise in K+
conductance  following  the  first  stimulus.     There   is   no
regenerative  response  to  the  second  stimulus because the K+
conductance is still elevated and the Na+ inactivation is  still
effective,  two  conditions  which make it difficult to get Na+
entry to exceed K+ exit.  It should be  recalled  that  the  two
conductances  are  on  scales  normalized  for  their respective
maxima which are quite different on an absolute scale.

        The  reason  for the absence of axes, scales, and labels
on this display is to emphasize that for  this  video  interface
the  CRT  is  entirely  separate  from  the  one  used  for  the
alphanumeric  displays  of  stimulus  parameters  and  output
displays.    It  is  necessary  to purchase separate hardware to
combine  the  two  circuits,  or  to  develop  special  software
routines  which  place  user-defined characters as points on the
screen.  Examples of these possibilities are included  elsewhere
in  this  chapter but their implementation is more detailed than
our  intended purpose.

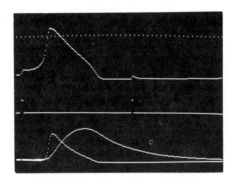

Fig.  12.3.  Plots of stimulus,
transmembrane  potential,  and
Na+  and  K+  conductances on a
256   by   240-point  graphics
interface used with S-100 based
microcomputers.     The     two
stimuli  are  identical but the
second  one  is  ineffective
because  of  the  continuing
permeability  to  K+  and  Na+
inactivation.

APPLE II GRAPHIC DISPLAYS

        The  Apple  II  has  integrated high-resolution graphics
which are useful for plotting the variables  as  a  function  of
time,  even  though  labels  must  be  supplied as user-defined
shapes.  The bottom of the graphics-mode screen can be  set  to
hold  four  lines  of  text  for time-axes labels, for scrolling

numerical values, or for running comments which are presented as
the variables are being plotted. Figure 12.4 is a photograph of
a CRT display taken from an Apple II which is simulating the
conditions for two stimuli in which the second one is large
enough to evoke a response. The relationship between the
different tracings is discussed in more detail in the next
section as a refractory period illustration.

Figure 12.4. A demonstration
of relative refractory period
illustrating the Apple II
graphic resolution. The two
bottom tracings are Na+ and K+
conductances normalized to
their respective maximum
values. When using a color
monitor it is possible to
assign different colors to
each of the plotted variables.

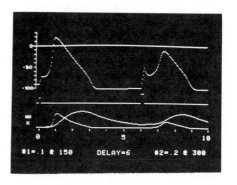

Before beginning the loop which displays and computes
the variables it is necessary to initialize the Apple II screen.
This computer has two high-resolution graphics mode commands,
HGR which gives 280 horizontal by 160 vertical points along with
4 lines of 40-characters at the bottom of the screen, and HGR2
which gives 280 horizontal by 196 vertical points. Either of
these commands clears the screen and prepares the computer to
accept vector and point-plotting commands to place axes and tic
marks.

As supplied there is no direct way of placing
alphanumeric characters within the graphics area. The
characters may be defined as a matrix of points or vectors and
saved in software subroutines. This approach is illustrated by
the small letters on the left of the display in Figure 12.4. In
this figure the axes and tics have been drawn using the vector
command HPLOT. The millisecond labels are in the top of the
four lines of text at the bottom of the screen. The bottom line
keeps the stimulus parameters in view.

Table 12.8 contains the subroutine which would be placed
at line 4000 to plot a response such as that shown in the
previous figure. This is based on the assumption that the DT
increment used was 1/25 msec so that 250 plotted points simulate
a time span of 10 msec. The sweeps in the subroutine begin at
X=25 and run through X=275 to define the 250 time increments.
The vertical dimension contains plots of four different
functions. The Applesoft BASIC high-resolution graphics command

is HPLOT X,Y to put a point at those coordinates on a screen intitialized with either the HGR or the HGR2 commands.

---

Table 12.8

A subroutine for plotting Hodgkin-Huxley variables on the Apple II microcomputer. The time axis starts at X=25 and each point corresponds to the resolution of DT. The ordinates contain vertical offsets and scale factors. The stimulus value is set according to the variable T. For plotting the tracings in different colors the individual HPLOT commands should be preceeded by an appropriate HCOLOR command.

```
4000 REM  -- APPLE II GRAPH OF ACTION POTENTIAL --
4010:
4020 X=25+(T/DT)                       (X stays same
4030 HPLOT X, 20-(MV/1.5)              (Millivolts
4040 HPLOT X, 150-(75*N*N*N*N)         (Normalized GK
4050 HPLOT X, 150-(75*M*M*M*H)         (Normalized GNa
4060 :
4070 REM  PLOT STIMULUS, IF ANY
4080 ST=0
4090 IF T< SD(1) THEN ST=SA(1)             (First?
4100 IF T=> DLY AND T< (DLY +SD(2)) THEN
        ST=ST+SA(2)                        (Second?
4110 HPLOT X, 110-(ST/20)                  (Stimulus
4120:
4130 IF X=> 275 THEN GOTO 4130         (Software halt
4140 RETURN
```

---

Line 4030 puts a dot at an x-coordinate corresponding to the time and at a Y location with 0 mv at 20 steps down on the screen. The variable MV is divided by 1.5 for scaling. Lines 4040 and 4050 place graphs of normalized Na+ and K+ conductances at Y=150 for a zero baseline. The number 75 provides amplitude scaling of the products of the dimensionless variables N, M, and H.

Lines 4080-4100 set a variable ST to the stimulus, depending upon the value of T. Line 4110 scales this amplitude and plots it above the Y=110 line. One method of terminating the simulation would be to put it in a software halt after 250 display increments as in line 4130. Of course there are many opportunities for plotting other variables. For example, in Figure 12.5 the plots of stimulus and conductances are replaced

with those of the three dimensionless variables, N, M, and H.
Here  the color option could be used to advantage to distinguish
between these overlapping tracings.  The one disadvantage is the
inconvenience  of placing alphanumeric characters in the graphic
area.  The major point to be made  is  that  the  Apple  II  has
reasonable graphic capabilities integrated into BASIC so that it
is convenient to use.

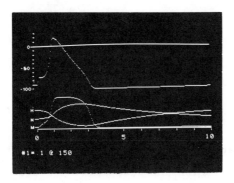

Fig. 12.5.  APPLE II plot of computed membrane potential and the
     three dimensionless variables following a stimulus  of  150
     units  lasting  0.1  msec.  Note the persistence of H and M
     long after the spike.

PROPERTIES OF EXCITATION

        Now that the BASIC programs for simulating  the  Hodgkin
and  Huxley  model on microcomputers has been given they will be
used to provide insight about the properties of excitation.  The
material is organized for lecture demonstrations with the choice
and format of computed variables being selected to emphasize the
salient  features  of  each  property.   Numerical  values  are
displayed as functions of time on CRT´s having 64 characters per
line.   The  computing increment is 0.01 msec and the increment
for output displays is adjusted to the rate  of  change  of  the
variables.   In  most  cases the graphic plots are computed and
displayed at time increments of 0.04 msec using the features  of
the Apple II as just described.  The speed of these computations
is tedious for use over extended periods but  for  demonstration
purposes  the  two  minutes  per  10  msec  sweep  does give the
instructor a chance for a running explanation.   Later  sections
in this chapter tell how to speed up these computations.

THRESHOLD

The initial changes in membrane conductances and currents near threshold are too small to be revealed by graphs so that it is more informative to present these as numerical values at successive time increments. Figure 12.6 shows the results of these computations for a subthreshold stimulus of 50 $\mu$amps/sq cm and a duration of 0.1 msec. The values in the first line correspond to the initial steady-state magnitudes as given in Table 12.3. The column headed MSC refers to the leakage current through a membrane channel having constant conductance. The initial total membrane current, which is very close to zero in this example, is a balance between the Na+ and leakage currents in and the K+ current out. Note that the resting K+ conductance is about 36 times that for Na+ but because of differences in the total electrochemical driving forces on these ions their respective currents are very similar in magnitude.

During the interval 0.0 to 0.1 msec the stimulating current transferred enough positive charge into the axon to depolarize the membrane by about 5 mv. This modifies the previously discussed first-order rate constants to new values, starting a change in membrane conductances to Na+ and K+, and also in the currents of these ions. Scan down each of the columns and note that K+ reaches a peak conductance near 3.6 msec while Na+ reaches its at about 1.2 msec. There are similar differences in the timing of the two currents.

Throughout the 4 msec time span the membrane currents are small with a gradual net outward loss of positive charge until the resting potential is reached again. It should be noted that the conductance changes last longer than the duration of the stimulus, evidence that the membrane is excitable. This response would not be sufficient to trigger a propagated impulse and is referred to as a "local response".

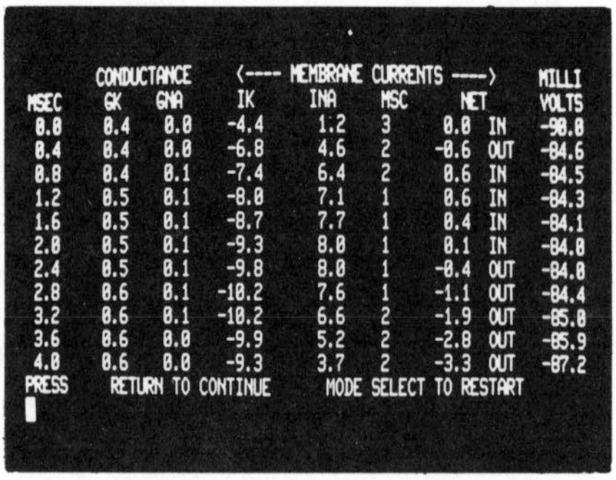

Fig. 12.6. Membrane conductances and currents for 4 msec after application of a subthreshold stimulus. The column labeled MSC is the leakage current which has constant conductance in the model. Units are as given in Table 12.3. Positive and inward currents are defined as the entry of positive charges into the axon.

| | CONDUCTANCE | | | <---- MEMBRANE CURRENTS ----> | | | MILLI |
|------|------|------|------|------|------|---------|--------|
| MSEC | GK | GNA | IK | INA | MSC | NET | VOLTS |
| 0.0 | 0.4 | 0.0 | -4.4 | 1.2 | 3 | 0.0 IN | -90.0 |
| 0.4 | 0.4 | 0.0 | -6.8 | 4.6 | 2 | -0.6 OUT | -84.6 |
| 0.8 | 0.4 | 0.1 | -7.4 | 6.4 | 2 | 0.6 IN | -84.5 |
| 1.2 | 0.5 | 0.1 | -8.0 | 7.1 | 1 | 0.6 IN | -84.3 |
| 1.6 | 0.5 | 0.1 | -8.7 | 7.7 | 1 | 0.4 IN | -84.1 |
| 2.0 | 0.5 | 0.1 | -9.3 | 8.0 | 1 | 0.1 IN | -84.0 |
| 2.4 | 0.5 | 0.1 | -9.8 | 8.0 | 1 | -0.4 OUT | -84.0 |
| 2.8 | 0.6 | 0.1 | -10.2 | 7.6 | 1 | -1.1 OUT | -84.4 |
| 3.2 | 0.6 | 0.1 | -10.2 | 6.6 | 2 | -1.9 OUT | -85.0 |
| 3.6 | 0.6 | 0.0 | -9.9 | 5.2 | 2 | -2.8 OUT | -85.9 |
| 4.0 | 0.6 | 0.0 | -9.3 | 3.7 | 2 | -3.3 OUT | -87.2 |
| PRESS | | RETURN TO CONTINUE | | | MODE SELECT TO RESTART | | |

The response to a stimulus of 150 μamps/sq cm of the same duration is a marked contrast. Figure 12.7 shows that starting from the same intitial steady-state this entry of positive charge depolarizes the membrane by about 15 mv. This is enough to start a regenerative process by which the entry of Na+ exceeds the entry of K+ so that the depolarization further enhances Na+ permeability. Note that the displayed time increments in this figure are 0.2 msec apart in order to reveal the rapid changes involved. At 0.4 msec the Na+ conductance is much greater than it is for the previous subthreshold example while the K+ conductances are very similar in the two situations. The increase in K+ current at 0.4 msec is not because of a conductance change but because the membrane electrical potential is further from the equilibrium value for this ion. Up to about 1 msec Na+ current far exceeds K+ so that its kinetics contributes to the shape of the rising part of the spike.

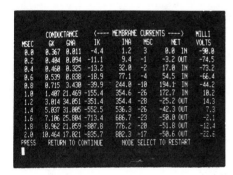

| | CONDUCTANCE | | | <---- MEMBRANE CURRENTS ----> | | | MILLI |
| MSEC | GK | GNA | IK | INA | MSC | NET | VOLTS |
| --- | --- | --- | --- | --- | --- | --- | --- |
| 0.0 | 0.367 | 0.011 | -4.4 | 1.2 | 3 | 0.0 IN | -90.0 |
| 0.2 | 0.404 | 0.094 | -11.1 | 9.4 | -1 | -3.2 OUT | -74.5 |
| 0.4 | 0.460 | 0.325 | -13.2 | 32.0 | -2 | 17.0 IN | -73.2 |
| 0.6 | 0.539 | 0.838 | -18.9 | 77.1 | -4 | 54.5 IN | -66.4 |
| 0.8 | 0.715 | 3.430 | -39.9 | 244.0 | -10 | 194.1 IN | -44.2 |
| 1.0 | 1.407 | 21.469 | -155.4 | 354.6 | -26 | 172.7 IN | 10.2 |
| 1.2 | 3.014 | 34.051 | -351.4 | 354.4 | -28 | -25.2 OUT | 14.3 |
| 1.4 | 5.037 | 31.005 | -552.5 | 536.3 | -26 | -42.3 OUT | 7.3 |
| 1.6 | 7.106 | 25.804 | -713.4 | 686.7 | -23 | -50.0 OUT | -2.1 |
| 1.8 | 8.962 | 21.059 | -807.8 | 776.2 | -20 | -51.8 OUT | -12.4 |
| 2.0 | 10.464 | 17.021 | -835.7 | 802.3 | -17 | -50.6 OUT | -22.6 |
| PRESS | RETURN TO CONTINUE | | | MODE SELECT TO RESTART | | | |

Figure 12.7. Computed membrane conductances and currents following a suprathreshold stimulus. The depolarization is sufficient to start a regenerative rise in Na+ conductance and current. Later the K+ current is greater, returning the membrane to its resting value.

The peak overshoot of the spike is between 1.0 and 1.2 msec at which time the K+ and leakage currents out begin to exceed the Na+ current in. A feature of this itemized accounting of the components involved is that it shows that K+ current increases by a factor of 100 times over resting though the conductance has increased by only ten times. This is because at the peak of the spike the total driving force on this ion is about ten times that at rest. Similarly the Na+ conductance has increased by a factor of 3,400 times over rest but the current is not similarly increased because the transmembrane electrical potential is near to the equilibrium potential for this ion.

Because the time of maximum Na+ conductance does not correspond to the time of minimum driving force upon Na+ there may be a small dip in the Na+ current near the peak of the spike. At this time the force upon the leakage ions is at a maximum but the current never becomes large because of the low value of the conductance for these ions. During the falling phase the Na+ and K+ currents are both much greater than at rest but the return of intracellular negativity requires only that K+ leave faster than Na+ enters.

Plots of these variables, as in Figure 12.4, give an overall view of the pattern of changes. In this figure the sequence and durations of the conductance changes can be correlated with the action potential but their relative magnitudes can not be compared. The initial rise in Na+ conductance, which is normalized for a maximum value of 120 units, corresponds to the time of rapid Na+ entry and depolarization. The slower, sustained rise in K+ conductance, normalized to a maximum of 36 units, favors the loss of K+ during repolarization. This phase lasts even after the potential returns to resting level, causing a period of hyperpolarization.

The three dimensionless variables used to quantitatively describe the conductance changes , are plotted in Figure 12.5. The short time constant of the Na+ activation variable M can be seen to follow the membrane potential changes reaching a plateau value near 1.0. But because the Na+ inactivation H is falling at this time the net action of the product of these variables is to lower membrane conductance to Na+ during the repolarization phase. The two variables M and H have long time constants and are still approaching their final values ten msec after the end of the stimulus. These persisting changes, along with the low value of M resulting from the hyperpolarization, contribute to the timing of the refractory period which follows a spike.

The kinetics of the conductance changes by which a membrane reaches threshold are strongly influenced by the rate and extent of the depolarization produced by the stimulus. The rapid depolarization by a large stimulus of short duration enhances the process of Na+ entry and the spike occurs soon after the stimulus is begun. At the other extreme the small depolarization produced by a weak stimulus has less influence upon the rate constants of the activation processes and there is a prolonged latency before the spike occurs, if it does.

Figure 12.8 illustrates this latency following a 0.1 msec stimulus of 53.5 μamps/sq cm magnitude. Figure 12.8A shows that for this small stimulus the Na+ conductance initially rises slowly so that for several milliseconds the total membrane currrent is small, though inward. It isn't until 4 msec that the Na+ current finally begins its rapid increase and the spike occurs. Figure 12.8B is a graphic display of the changes in membrane potentials and absolute values of conductances over a 10 msec time span. Students enjoy making a game out of finding the exact stimulus which will give a full spike but, with a slight reduction in stimulus, produces only a local response.

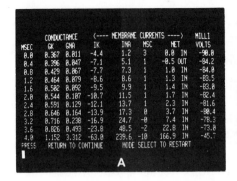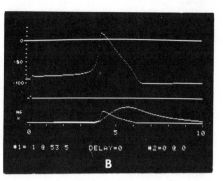

| MSEC | CONDUCTANCE GK | GNA | IK | INA | MSC | NET | MILLI VOLTS |
|------|------|------|------|------|------|------|------|
| 0.0 | 0.367 | 0.011 | -4.4 | 1.2 | 3 | 0.0 IN | -90.0 |
| 0.4 | 0.396 | 0.047 | -7.1 | 5.1 | 1 | -0.5 OUT | -84.2 |
| 0.8 | 0.429 | 0.067 | -7.7 | 7.3 | 1 | 1.0 IN | -84.0 |
| 1.2 | 0.464 | 0.079 | -8.6 | 8.6 | 1 | 1.3 IN | -83.5 |
| 1.6 | 0.502 | 0.092 | -9.5 | 9.9 | 1 | 1.4 IN | -83.0 |
| 2.0 | 0.544 | 0.107 | -10.7 | 11.5 | 1 | 1.7 IN | -82.4 |
| 2.4 | 0.591 | 0.129 | -12.1 | 13.7 | 1 | 2.3 IN | -81.6 |
| 2.8 | 0.646 | 0.164 | -13.9 | 17.3 | 0 | 3.7 IN | -80.4 |
| 3.2 | 0.716 | 0.238 | -16.9 | 24.7 | -0 | 7.4 IN | -78.3 |
| 3.6 | 0.826 | 0.493 | -23.8 | 48.5 | -2 | 22.8 IN | -73.0 |
| 4.0 | 1.152 | 3.312 | -63.0 | 239.6 | -10 | 166.9 IN | -45.7 |

PRESS RETURN TO CONTINUE    MODE SELECT TO RESTART

A

#1= 1 @ 53.5     DELAY=0     #2=0 @ 0

B

Fig. 12.8. Latency of the response following a threshold value of stimulus. A) The net membrane current stays small for several milliseconds until at 4.0 msec the Na+ entry finally becomes regenerative. B) Note the delay in conductance changes and in membrane voltage rise. There is a graded progression of latencies depending upon stimulus magnitude. The conductances in this graph are plotted on absolute scales.

## TEMPORAL SUMMATION

Because the changes in membrane conductances outlast the duration of subthreshold stimuli it is possible to accumulate the effects of two of these applied in rapid succession. This is illustrated in Figure 12.9 where two stimuli of 40 µamps/sq cm and 0.1 msec duration are separated by about 1 msec. A student exercise could consider the first stimulus as a conditioning one and the second as a test stimulus for mapping out the temporal change in excitability following a subthreshold stimulus. Note that in this figure the absolute values of sodium and potassium conductances are plotted to the same scale.

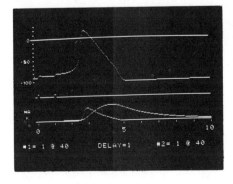

#1= 1 @ 40     DELAY=1     #2=.1 @ 40

Fig. 12.9. Temporal summation of two subthreshold stimuli. Either one alone will not evoke a regenerative response but if sufficiently close to one another their effects will be additive.

ANODE-BREAK EXCITATION

        Graphic   simulations   can   be   used   to   advantage   to
appreciate   the   fact   that   excitation   can   follow releasing a
membrane from a hyperpolarized state.  The name  of  anode-break
excitation arises from the fact that a "shock" is felt under the
anode when the current is interrupted.  The  same  mechanism  is
used   to   explain   "inhibition   rebound"   where   excitability is
increased after a period of inhibition.  Figure 12.10 is a  plot
of a membrane potential initially equilibrated at a steady-state
value of -105 mv and then released from this  condition  at  the
start  of  the  simulation.  In subsequent increments of time the
membrane currents are determined by the  respective  forces  and
conductances  upon the individual ions.  There is no stimulating
current.

        In   this   figure   the   stimulus and conductance tracings
have  been  replaced  by  plots  of  the   three   dimensionless
parameters  N,  M,  and  H.  If these tracings are compared with
those  in  Figure  12.5  obtained  for  an  initial  steady-state
voltage  of -90 mv it can be seen that the hyperpolarization has
changed each of these variables drastically.   The  variable  N
which   determines   K+ conductance is much lower, reducing the K+
current  to  much  lower than its normal resting value.   The  Na+
inactivation  variable  H,  which  is  inherently  slow, is much
greater.   Likewise   in   the  hyperpolarized state there   is
increased  driving  force  upon  the  Na+  and less upon the K+.
These altered forces and conductances favor  the  entry  of  Na+
over the exit of K+ so that it is possible to get a regenerative
process starting from the hyperpolarized state.

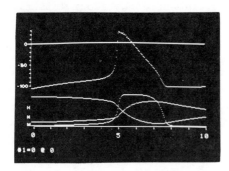

Figure  12.10.  The changes in
voltage and variables after  a
steady-state hyperpolarization
at -105 mv.  The high value of
H and the low value of N favor
the entry of Na+ over the exit
of  K+.   The  Na+  activation
variable M reaches  a  plateau
near  1.0  during  the  spike.
Other  variables  are  plotted to
the same scale.

ACCOMMODATION

        A  stimulus  of  low  amplitude  and continuing duration
might be expected to eventually elicit a response.   Instead  it
actually can reduce the excitablity to a standard test stimulus.
Membranes have the useful property of adapting or  accommodating

to persisting stimuli.    Figure   12.11   illustrates   this   using
scales which differ from those used in the other plots.    In this
figure the voltage scale is amplified to show a range of -90    to
-80   mv   and   the absolute values of K+ and Na+ conductances are
plotted to the same scale.    The   conditioning   stimulus   is   1.5
μamps/sq   cm   for   a   duration   of 8 msec.    Initially there is a
gradual depolarization as would be expected from the entrance of
this positive charge, however lagging behind this voltage change
is an increase in K+ conductance.

        At   about   5 msec the membrane conductance has increased
so much that K+   is   able   to   leak   out   faster   than   the   1.5
conditioning   current   can enter so that there is actually a net
loss in intracellular positive charge until the test stimulus is
applied   at   8   msec.    At that time the 100 unit test stimulus,
which   is   normally   above   threshold,   produces   a   membrane
depolarization   of   about   10 mv.   However this time the high K+
conductance and Na+ deactivation make it more difficult   to   get
Na+   to enter faster than K+ leaves.    The threshold for the test
signal has been elevated significantly.

Fig.   12.11.   Membrane voltage
and conductance changes   during
a    constant   stimulus   of   low
amplitude           demonstrating
accommodation.       The   voltage
scale is amplified to show   -90
to   -80   mv; absolute values of
K+   and   Na+   conductances   are
plotted to the same scale.    The
constant       inward       current
initially     depolarizes     the
membrane but as K+   conductance
increases there is eventually a
net loss of positive charge.

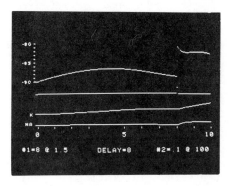

REFRACTORY PERIOD

        The explanation for the refractory   period   following   a
spike   is   contained   in several figures.    In Figure 12.3, where
two identical stimuli were separated by 5 msec, it can   be   seen
that   the   effect   of   the   second   stimulus   is   limited to the
depolarization brought about by the transfer of positive   charge
into   the   axon.   A partial explanation is seen in the fact that
at the time of this stimulus the membrane K+   conductance   still
remains   elevated   after   the   first one.   This means that it is
then difficult to get Na+ to enter more rapidly than K+ exits.

        By   waiting   until   a   later   time   and   using   a   larger
stimulus it is possible to elicit a second response though it is
modified   in form.    Figure 12.4 shows   a depolarization   by   the

second stimulus which is sufficient to start a regenerative
response. However, the kinetics of the Na+ conductance changes
are markedly reduced so that the rate of rise and extent of the
spike is considerably different from that following the first
stimulus.

The time course for the recovery of excitability
following an action potential can be appreciated from the plots
of the dimensionless variables in Figure 12.5. Na+
inactivation, denoted by H, reduces the Na+ conductance for
several milliseconds. During the hyperpolarization phase the
Na+ activation variable M is low so that these two factors
reduce the Na+ permeability to values even less than at rest.
Following the peak of the spike the K+ activation variable N is
elevated and quantitatively describes sustained high permeablity
to K+ at that time. These two factors combine to make it more
difficult to get Na+ to enter faster than K+ exits. In addition
to these membrane conductance changes the driving forces are
drastically different near the peak of the spike. At this time
the electric voltage difference across the membrane nearly
balances the Na+ concentration gradient and the total
electrochemical gradient for K+ is at a maximum. These
conditions would also contribute to the difficulty in getting a
regenerative entry of Na+ during the absolute refractory period.

The duration of the refractory period limits the rate at
which information can be carried by an axon. A common teaching
exercise is to map out the return of excitabiliy following a
normal action potential. This can be done easily through
simulation by setting the delay to different values and
adjusting the test stimulus to find threshold intensity.
Furthermore, this process can be automated in a computer loop
using a constant second stimulus but changing only the delay
until its initiation. This demonstration can be run on
lecture-hall monitors during between-class breaks or in hallway
display cabinets for additional exposure.

CONSTANT STIMULATING CURRENT

Axons carry information in terms of the number of action
potentials occurring per unit of time. Simulation can show that
constant inward current of sufficient amplitude will elicit
repeated responses at a frequency which is a function of the
stimulus amplitude. Figure 12.12 has two simulations at two
different stimulus amplitudes over a time span of 50 msec.
These are obtained by plotting every fifth computed value and so
take proportionately longer to execute. That on the left, where
the amplitude is 15 units, has 4 spikes during the 50 msec; that
on the right, with an amplitude of 50 units, has 6 spikes in the
same time span. This can be understood in terms of the more
rapid depolarization effected by the stronger stimulus.

Note the differences in the shapes and sizes of the action potentials. The first stimulus in each sweep starts from a steady-state condition and gives a full voltage swing but subsequent spikes are diminished because of the residual changes in conductance after an excitation. This is particularly evident in the tracings of the Na+ conductance at the bottom which show larger initial changes in each and with amplitudes reduced according to the time since the last excitation. Nevertheless the computed spikes would be large enough to be propagated in a normal axon.

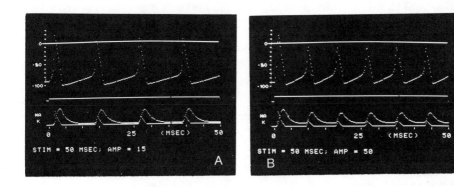

Fig. 12.12.  Repeated spikes resulting from constant stimuli of two different amplitudes. The total sweep is 50 msec in these figures.  A)  For a value of 15 units there are 4 spikes within 50 msec.  B) For a value of 50 units there are 6 spikes in the same time. In both cases the initial responses are larger because of the larger Na+ conductance changes; subsequent responses are reduced because of the lasting nature of the Na+ inactivation and K+ activation.


OTHER PROPERTIES

A favorite neurophysiology teaching demonstration is to plot out the reciprocal relationship between the duration of a stimulus and the threshold value. This information is used to determine the rheobase, a quantity which is significantly greater if a muscle is the tissue being excited than if a nerve is the site of excitation.  As a first approximation the product of stimulating current and duration required to transfer the membrane from resting potential to threhold is a constant. However at long durations, when there is time for accommodative loss of K+, it requires more charge in the stimulus. At very low amplitudes it may be impossible to overcome this accommodation as is seen in Figure 12.11.

Before assigning a class to undertake this exercise on a microcomputer equipped with the routines given so far the instructor should be aware of the following pitfalls. First, to get several points on the relationship takes an unrealistic amount of time at two minutes per complete simulation. Secondly, because of the finite integration intervals used the computed charge transferred by a stimulus is going to be in multiples of DT. This give serious inconsistencies at short stimulus durations. For example, if DT is 0.04 as used in the graphic simulations, changing the stimulus duration from 0.05 to 0.99 msec may have no influence upon the threshold current, a point which will be confusing to students. The answer to both of these problems is to design a simulation specifically for this exercise in which the values of DT are very small and have the process terminate without waiting for the full spike. Also see the discussion of computation speed on page 188.

Hodgkin's and Huxley's voltage-dependent rate constants were standardized to the same temperature by using a temperature coefficient of 3 and scaling them to 6.3 degrees centigrade. Thus it is possible to do an exercise looking at the membrane responses at warmer temperatures by multiplying the rate coefficients by a suitable factor. For example, the constant AN, the rate of potassium OFF to ON states as defined in the subroutine given previously, would be replaced by

$$AN = AN * 3^{((TEMP-6.3)/10)}$$

where the variable TEMP is the temperature to be used for the simulation. Thus at a value of TEMP=16.3 the rate constants would each be multiplied by a factor of 3.

Figure 12.13 illustates the nature of the Na+ and K+ conductance changes for voltage clamp conditions, similar to those found experimentally by Hodgkin and Huxley. A step change from resting potential to -30 mv initiates the rapid rise in Na+ conductance followed by the slower, sustained rise in K+ conductance. The absolute values of conductances are plotted on the same scale. Upon return to the resting potential there is no change in Na+ permeability but this property of K+ begins its slow fall at that time.

It is possible to observe the differing kinetics of these two membrane properties for different amounts of depolarization. Initial hyperpolarized conditions demonstrate a low peak in GK, the explanation for excitation at an anode break. Initial steady-state depolarization attenuates the Na+ kinetics and enhances K+ responses, reducing excitability. The only programming change required for this exercise is to place a command in the iteration loop which constantly sets MV to the clamped value regardless of what net current has been transferred during the integration interval.

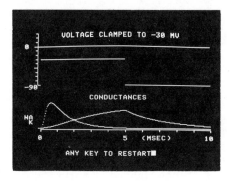

Figure 12.13. NA+ and K+ conductance changes following a step change in membrane potential to a clamped value. The Hodgkin and Huxley equations empirically fit curves such as these for different amounts of depolarization.

## COMPUTATION METHODS

The programs given in the previous sections of this chapter have been written in BASIC with considerable documentation and have used simple Euler methods of integrating the dimensionless variables and the transmembrane potential. This has been done for clarity of presentation and for the most likely microcomputer configurations to be used by the audience of this book. However, such a presentation does not make use of the full computation speed and accuracy possible for microcomputer simulations. This section makes some general comments about the possibilities for improving both of these facets using different software. The final section discusses a hardware method of improving computation speed.

The topic of the accuracy of iterative integrations of differential equations is a very technical one. When the analytical solution for an integration is known it is possible to measure the accuracy of a given method of digital integration, but for a system of simultaneous nonlinear differential equations the evaluation of accuracy does not come so easily. Instead the "true" solution is found experimentally by taking successively smaller integration steps until the solution becomes independent of the size of these steps.

For teaching purposes, when speed is a major consideration, the criterion of accuracy can be relaxed to that showing no unphysiological responses. Using the Euler method the author has found that steps of greater than 0.05 msec introduce extraneous oscillations just after the peak of the spike. The excitation following prolonged hyperpolarization is particularly sensitive to this instability. Even at this step size there is the previously mentioned error in that the stimulus duration actually realized is in multiples of DT, not

necessarily the value entered by the operator. In circumstances
where this error is serious it is possible to have the program
adjust the amplitude of the stimulus so that the total charge
delivered by the stimulus is corrrect.

SPEED

        A previous chapter mentioned that microprocessors can be
run at a wide range of clock frequencies, the rate at which
individual machine code commands are executed. There are many
S-100 bus central processing units (CPU's) which use 4 MHz
versions of the 8080/8085/Z-80 microprocessors. This is clearly
a speed advantage. The 6802 microprocessor, used in the PET and
the APPLE microcomputers, has a "look ahead" feature which
increases its effective computation speed. However, when most
physiologists purchase a microcomputer for simulation they are
likely to seek an integrated system in which the microprocessor
speed is not the overriding consideration. Software
optimization of speed and accuracy are important for any
hardware configuration.

        The conveniences of an interactive interpreter-driven
language such as BASIC are achieved at the cost of speed. The
use of compiler-driven BASIC, FORTRAN, or Pascal languages can
speed up iterative computation loops by a factor of three to ten
times. These forms of high-level languages, which utilize
efficient machine coded instructions at the time of execution,
are becoming more widely available for microcomputers and are
certainly good investments for serious simulation work.
Nevertheless, BASIC plays the important function of getting the
benefits of instructional simulation into the hands of teachers
who have minimal interest in computers and programming. Some
computation or display feature can be changed easily in a BASIC
program during a lecture demonstration while few people would be
brave enough to recompile a FORTRAN program in front of a class
of 100 impatient students.

        Speed is not an important consideration for initializing
the simulation where entries by the operator are the limiting
factor. Any saving in time in the iteration loop becomes
significant when it is multiplied by the number of times the
loop is traversed during a simulation. The author has divided
this loop, outlined in general form in Table 12.1, into three
major steps and has compared each of these for the three
prototype microcomputers. Though there were minor differences
between the three computers the significant finding is that
about 50% of the time is spent on evaluating the rate constants;
slightly more than 25% is on updating the variables; and
slightly less than 25% is on graphic displays of the variables.
Clearly the large number of exponentials in the subroutine of
Table 12.4 consume considerable computation time. Ways of
reducing this time are considered later.

The Apple II, which uses a 5-byte floating point format for 9-digit precision, takes 0.56 sec per iteration which includes plotting four variables. For a total of 250 points at DT=0.04 msec this computes and displays a 10 msec sweep in 140 seconds on the Apple II and in 165 seconds on the SOL, an S-100 bus computer. A TRS-80 routine which displays only one variable requires 0.72 sec per iteration. There are a number of ways to make small improvements in the timing of all of these, such as deleting comment statements, using variables instead of computed constants, and by moving the subroutines into the iteration loop itself. Dr. George Beeler kindly has pointed out to the author that the number of exponentials in Table 12.4 could be reduced from six to four by defining values of EXP(1), EXP(2.5), and EXP(3) as constants. These can be used as products with a single EXP(V+10) in lines 3080, 3100, and 3110. This reduces the Apple II time for 250 points from 140 seconds to 130 seconds. Many other housekeeping changes, such as eliminating the time to call subroutines and dropping out the tests for division by zero, reduces the time from 130 to 120 seconds.

For computers with sufficient memory it is possible to eliminate the exponential computations entirely during each iteration by using a lookup table as mentioned by Hodgkin and Huxley in their original paper. Upon starting the simulation for the first time arrays are established with values of AN(I), BN(I), AM(I), BM(I), AH(I), and BH(I) at 1 mv increments of the membrane voltage. The range of these increments covers the expected limits from hyperpolarization to the peak of the spike. Upon each iteration the index I is set according to the present voltage and the dimensionless variables N, M, and H are updated with the appropriate rate constants as before except these are now subscripted. It takes about 30 seconds to initialize this array, a time which can be shared with text panels giving the objectives and instructions for the simulation exercise.

Alternatively, the array, which occupies about 6K bytes of memory, can be loaded as data from the disk within a few seconds. Once the subscripted rate constants are in place the time for the iteration loop to compute and display each point is cut in half. For clarity of presentation the Applesoft BASIC program in the Chapter Appendix calculates the exponentials as they are used, even though this is a time-consuming approach.

ACCURACY

The major sources of inaccuracy in digital simulation of the Hodgkin and Huxley equations arise in the integration of the first-order differential equations which describe the changes in the dimensionless parameters, and in updating the membrane voltage. Professionals commonly have used Runge-Kutta integration schemes which evaluate several derivatives to find

the best value to be used to update the time-dependent
variables. This gives considerable accuracy but at a marked
reduction in speed. Moore and Ramon (1974) did an experimental
study in which they compared several alternative methods of
integrating these equations in regard to the latency and
accuracy of the waveform. They found that the major source of
error is an overestimating of the incremental changes in the
variable M, the measure of Na+ activation which has the shortest
time constant of the three variables. They found that the
simple Euler method, when modified for better estimates of
changes in M, gives accuracy approaching the Runga-Kutta method
but with significant savings in speed.

One method of finding better estimates of the changes in
N, M, and H during the integration intervals is described in the
paper by Moore and Ramon, and used in simulations by Rush and
Larsen (1978). Rather than assuming these variables to be
constants during the duration of the increment DT, as is the
case in the Euler method, it is assumed that they change
exponentially following a path which can be calculated from
known information. The evaluation of the value of these
dimensionless variables at the end of the integration step
involves an additional exponential which adds to the computation
time but which does not change the shape of the spike at the
graphic resolution being used here. In the case of the
ventricular action potential discussed in the next chapter,
inclusion of this correction does permit using a longer
integration interval with a net gain in speed.

The modification of changes in M which Moore and Ramon
used requires minimal computation time and can be included as a
single statement. The reader is referred to their paper for a
discussion of the justification of this correction. Here it is
achieved by the simple expedient of inserting the line

        5035 DM = DM * (1 - (2.1 * DT))

into the subroutine given in Table 8.5. This replaces the
change in the rate constant AM as computed in line 5030 with a
slightly different value depending upon the value of DT and a
constant 2.1. This correction factor can be considered as the
first term in a series expansion of the exponential change
mentioned in the previous paragraph.

Another approach to optimizing speed vs accuracy
compromises is to adjust the integration step size according to
the rate of change of the variable with the shortest time
constant. After the spike the Na+ activation variable changes
very slowly so that the kinetics are dominated by the slower N
and H variables. Minimal error is introduced if the DT is
increased when the stimulus is not present and the rate of

change of voltage, or some other combination of variables, falls below a selected minimum. Figure 12.14 shows a plot in which the integration step size is increased to 0.16 msec after the spike. For exercises in which the primary interest is upon threshold events this speeds up the overall simulation time to values as low as 35 seconds for the 10 msec sweep time. In order to handle the variable sizes of DT it is necessary to change the statement for setting the abcissa in the display subroutine to the following

     4020 X = 25 + 250 * (T/10)

in which T/10 corresponds to the fraction of the total span of 250 points in the sweep. In this figure the plot of the MV variable is made continuous by use of the HPLOT command as a vector connecting successive values. The other variables are displayed as separated points to emphasize where the integration step changed size to a larger value.

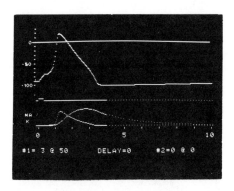

FIGURE 12.14. A simulation which increases the integration step size when the rates of change are reduced. This expedient, along with a lookup table for the rate constants, can compute and display a single spike within 35 seconds using Applesoft BASIC routines. Points of the voltage plot are connected by using the HPLOT command as a vector.


NUMERICAL PROCESSOR ROUTINES

     Up to this point the programs for simulating the axon membrane potentials have been written in BASIC, the language most commonly used with microcomputers. These run slowly because they use an interpreter and because the floating point mathematical subroutines consist of a large number of operations. The minimum time for generating a 10-msec sweep with usuable accuracy is approximately one minute, a discouraging wait not conducive to full exploration of all of the ramifications of the model. Chapter 4 discusses a numerical processor chip which can execute the common mathematical functions upon issue of a single machine code command. Futhermore, once started this chip proceeds independently freeing up the microprocessor for other operations. Such a hardware enhancement has the capability of increasing simulation

speeds by a factor of ten times providing a full action
potential within about ten seconds.

As the scientific applications for microcomputers are
developed the advantages of the Am-9511 Arithmetic Processor
Unit (APU) floating point chip are being recognized. BASIC
routines run the action potential simulation about twice as fast
if the software floating point routines are replaced with this
hardware version. Chapter 4 names a manufacturer who has an APU
interface card for S-100 bus microcomputers and a version of
Micosoft FORTRAN which uses its features. The realization of a
factor of ten increase in speed requires that the "number
crunching" aspects of the simulation be written using editors
and assembly language programming. This is a tedious process
but once done for a given machine its advantages can be shared
by many provided that there is a way to transport the software
between the computers at different institutions.

The author has written machine language subroutines,
based upon the 8080 microprocessor and the AM-9511 numererical
processor chip, which perform the graphic simulations rapidly.
He has used these for teaching demonstrations and student study
exercises on both the TRS-80 and a S-100 bus microcomputer. The
graph in Figure 12.2 is plotted on a TRS-80 in 10 seconds; that
in Figure 12.15, using a Matrox display interface, requires 8
seconds. These routines can be modified for the 6802
microprocessor used in the Apple II in order to take full
advantage of its integrated graphics capabilities. The full
machine language programs are too detailed to be of general
interest so the balance of this chapter gives the guidelines for
implementing the numerical processor subroutines.

Figure 12.15. Machine-language
simulation generated within 8
seconds on an S-100 based
microcomputer. This uses a
numerical processor chip and a
240 by 256 point graphics
interface board. The same
speed is realized on either the
TRS-80 or the Apple II with
appropriate hardware additions.

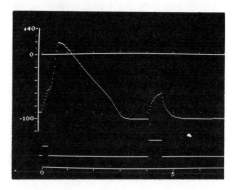

The reader is referred to Chapter 4 for a discussion of
the numerical processor chip and the software requirements for
its use. The general approach is to use BASIC to ask for the
stimulus parameters and to place them in a buffer area in the
format appropriate for the numerical processor's floating point

operations.  Once this is done control is transferred from BASIC
to  the  machine  language  routines which perform the iteration
loop.  A memory location is  set  up  to  count  the  number  of
iterations.  The individual operations within the iteration loop
peform the same functions as those in the BASIC routine of Table
12.1  except that they are performed in machine language code as
produced by an assembler.    Pointers  are  set  to  the  memory
addresses  of  numerical  constants,  stimulus  parameters,  or
computed variables.  Then subroutines are  called  which  "push"
these 4-byte floating point numbers onto the numerical processor
"stack".  As soon as one  or  more  these  arguments  have  been
placed on the processor stack the numerical operation command is
issued.  After the function is evaluated the result is  "popped"
from the stack into the buffer area at a labeled address.

        The process of  implementing  these  operations  can  be
considered manual compilation of a list of BASIC statements.  As
an illustration consider how the author implemented line 3120 of
Table  12.4  in  8080  assembly language.  This is the statement
which set the rate constant AH according to the current  voltage
V,

        3120 AH = 0.07 * EXP(V/20).

The  steps  are  similar  to  those in a reverse Polish notation
calculator.  The present voltage V is pushed onto the APU stack,
followed  by  the  constant  20.    With  these arguments in the
numerical processor  the  command  to  execute  the  exponential
function  is  given.    Then the constant 0.07 is pushed onto the
stack  and  the  floating  point  multiply  command  is  issued.
Finally this result is popped from the APU stack and placed into
the buffer area at the location labeled AH.  Thus a sequence  of
machine  language  calls  is  set  up following the logic of the
BASIC program.  After the iteration loop  counter  is  satisfied
control is returned back to the BASIC program which asks for the
next stimulus parameters.

        Table  12.9  gives  the portion of the assembler listing
which performs the function of the BASIC statement in line 3120.
In line 6010 the HL register pair of the 8080 is set to point to
the location of the variable VOLTS in the  buffer  area.    Line
6020  calls  a  subroutine  which  pushes the four bytes of that
variable onto the APU stack one byte at  a  time.    In  order  to
reduce  the number of constants stored in the buffer the integer
20 is put into the 8080 accumulator in line 6030  and  then  the
subroutine PUSHACC floats this and pushes it onto the APU stack.
There are now two arguments on the  stack  so  subroutine  FDIV
causes  the  AM-9511 to do a floating point divide, leaving V/20
on the stack.  This is followed by  a  call  to  the  subroutine
which  uses  this  result  as  the  argument for the exponential
function.  It is in this step where the the numerical  processor
provides  significant  savings  in computation time  over  software

floating point subroutines. Lines 6070 to 6090 move the 4-byte
values for the constant 0.07 onto the stack and then do a
floating point multiply. Finally the 8080 registers HL are used
as pointers to the buffer address for saving the computed value
of AH and the subroutine POPFLT pops its 4-byte representation
into that address.

---

### Table 12.9

Assembly language listing for 8080 microprocessor and
Am-9511 numerical processor which perform the
functions of line 3120 in the BASIC subroutine in
Table 12.4. The microprocessor register pairs are set
as pointers to floating point variables. Subroutines
are called which push these variables onto the 9511
stack, issue the command for a mathematical operation,
and then pop the result from the stack into the buffer
area.

```
6000  ;CALCULATE AH=0.07 * EXP(V/20)
6010     LXI      H,VOLTS         ;HL POINTS TO VOLTS
6020     CALL     PUSHFLT         ;VOLTS ONTO STACK
6030     MVI      A,20            ;INT 20 INTO ACCUM
6040     CALL     PUSHACC         ;FLOAT AND PUSH 20
6050     CALL     FDIV            ;APU= (V/20)
6060     CALL     FEXP            ;APU= EXP(V/20)
6070     LXI      H,P07           ;HL POINTS TO 0.07
6080     CALL     PSHFLT          ;APU= .07;EXP(V/20)
6090     CALL     FMUL            ;APU= .07*EXP(V/20)
6100     LXI      H,AH            ;HL POINTS TO AH
6110     CALL     POPFLT          ;POP AH INTO BUFFER
```

---

If one starts with a functioning BASIC program the
machine language portions can be written and debugged in logical
stages. For the 8080 microprocessor its register pairs HL, BC,
and DE are used to store pointers to addresses of variables in
the buffer area. Communication between the AM-9511 and the
microprocessor is achieved via the latter's I/O ports as
identified by the interfacing circuitry. For the 6802
microprocessor in the Apple II the pointers are stored in memory
locations and the I/O ports are specific memory locations
assigned for peripheral devices. Since the Am-9511 uses 4-byte
floating point and Applesoft BASIC uses five bytes there is a
loss in precision in using the numerical processor. This is not
a noticeable limitation for this application.

# REFERENCES

Fitzhugh, R.: Thresholds and plateaus in the Hodgkin-Huxley nerve equations. J. Gen. Physiol. 43:867-896 (1960).

Fitzhugh, R.: Anodal excitation in the Hodgkin-Huxley nerve model. Biophys. J. 16:209-226 (1976).

Goldman, L., and C. L. Schauf: Quantitative description of sodium and potassium currents and computed action potentials in Myxicola giant axons. J. Gen. Physiol. 61:361-384 (1973).

Hodgkin, A. L., and A. F. Huxley: A quantitative description of membrane current and its application to conduction and excitation in nerves. J. Physiol. 117:500-544 (1952).

Moore, J. W., and F. Ramon: On numerical integration of the Hodgkin and Huxley equations for a membrane action potential. J. Theor. Biol. 45:249-273 (1974).

Randall, J. E. Teaching by simulation with personal computers. Physiol. Teacher, Physiologist 21:37-40 (1978).

Rush, S., and H. Larsen: A practical algorithm for solving dynamic membrane equations. IEEE Trans. of Biomed. Engr. BME-25:389-392 (1978).

Stewart, P. A. The action potential. Ch.8 in Engineering Principals in Physiology. Vol. I. J. H. U. Brown and D. S. Gann, Eds. New York: Academic Press (1973).

# CHAPTER APPENDIX

The following three pages contain a listing of an Apple II program which follows the general plan presented in this chapter. This arrangement serves a teaching purpose for the reader but it takes an excessive amount of time to run. For example, the exponentials are evaluated as they are used, an operation which consumes a significant amount of time. Also the routines for placing labels in the high-resolution graphics area are omitted. Note that the absolute conductances of sodium and potassium are plotted in the subroutine at line 4000 whereas their normalized values are displayed in some of the figures.

```
10   REM   AXON ACTION POTENTIAL
20   REM        HODGKIN AND HUXLEY
30   REM         J. PHYSIOL. 117:500 (1952)
40   REM   THIS VERSION COMPUTES EXP() AS USED
50   REM                    ABSOLUTE CONDUCTANCES
60   REM                    NO ORDINATE LABELS
70 :
80 :
100  REM  ->GET STIM; SET STEADY-STATE VALUES<-
150  TEXT : HOME : REM CLEAR SCREEN
200  GOSUB 2000: REM --GET STIMULUS PARAMETERS
300  T = 0:DT = 1 / 25
400  MV =  - 90
500  GOSUB 3000: REM --SET ALPHA,BETA
600  GOSUB 3200: REM --S-S N,M,H
700  GOSUB 3500: REM --S-S G, I´S
710  GOSUB 6000: REM --AXES,LABELS
720 :
730 :
800  REM  ->LOOPS HERE EACH ITERATION<-----
900  GOSUB 4000: REM --DISPLAY VARIABLES
1000  GOSUB 3000: REM --SET ALPHA,BETA
1100  GOSUB 5000: REM --UPDATE G´S
1200  GOSUB 5500: REM --UPDATE I´S
1300  GOSUB 5700: REM --UPDATE VOLTS
1400 T = T + DT
1500  GOTO 800: REM   NEXT ITERATION ------>
1600 :
1610 :
2000 : REM  -> GET STIMULUS VALUES <-
2001  TEXT : HOME : VTAB 5: HTAB 5
2002  PRINT "ENTER STIMULUS PARAMETERS"
2003  PRINT : PRINT
2100  INPUT "STIM #1   ";SA(1)
2200  INPUT "  DURAT  ";SD(1)
2300  INPUT "DELAY     ";DLY
2400  INPUT "STIM #2  ";SA(2)
2500  INPUT "  DURAT  ";SD(2)
2600  RETURN
2700 :
3000  REM  -> RATE CONSTANTS FOR VOLTS <-
3020 V =  - MV - 90
3030  IF V + 25 = 0 THEN V =  - 25.1: REM   AVOID 1/0
3040  IF V + 10 = 0 THEN V =  - 10.1
3050 :
3060 BN = 0.125 *  EXP (V / 80)
3070 BM = 4 *  EXP (V / 18)
3080 BH = 1 / ( EXP ((V + 30) / 10) + 1)
3100 AN = 0.01 * (V + 10) / ( EXP ((V + 10) / 10) - 1)
3110 AM = 0.1 * (V + 25) / ( EXP ((V + 25) / 10) - 1)
3120 AH = 0.07 *  EXP (V / 20)
3140  RETURN
```

```
3200  REM  -> STEADY-STATE VARIABLES <-
3210 N = AN / (AN + BN)
3220 M = AM / (AM + BM)
3230 H = AH / (AH + BH)
3240  RETURN
3250 :
3500  REM  -> INITIAL G'S, I'S  <-
3520 GK = 36 * N * N * N * N
3530 GNA = 120 * M * M * M * H
3550 IK = GK * (V - 12)
3560 INA = GNA * (V + 115)
3570 IL = 0.3 * (V + 10.6)
3590 IT = IK + INA + IL
3610  RETURN
3999 :
4000  REM   APPLE II GRAPHICS DISPLAY
4020 X = 25 + (T / DT)
4025  REM   OR X=25+250*(T/10)
4030  HPLOT X,20 - (MV / 1.5)
4040  HPLOT X,150 - 1.5 * GK: REM   (ABSOLUTE CONDUCTANCE)
4050  HPLOT X,150 - 1.5 * GNA
4070  REM   STIMULUS, IF ANY
4080 ST = 0
4090  IF T < SD(1) THEN ST = SA(1)
4100  IF T = > DLY AND T < (DLY + SD(2)) THEN ST = ST + SA(2)
4110  HPLOT X,110 - (ST / 20)
4130  IF X = > 275 THEN  GOTO 4130: REM   (SOFTWARE HALT)
4140  RETURN
4199 :
5000  REM  -> UPDATE CONDUCTANCES <-
5020 DN = AN * (1 - N) - BN * N
5030 DM = AM * (1 - M) - BM * M
5040 DH = AH * (1 - H) - BH * H
5060 N = N + DN * DT
5070 M = M + DM * DT
5080 H = H + DH * DT
5100 GK = 36 * N * N * N * N
5110 GNA = 120 * M * M * M * H
5130  RETURN
5140 :
5500  REM  -> NEW CURRENTS <-
5520 IK = GK * (V - 12)
5530 INA = GNA * (V + 115)
5540 IL = 0.3 * (V + 10.6)
5550 IT = IK + IN + IL
5560 :
5570  REM   IS THERE A STIMULUS TO ADD?
5580  IF T < SD(1) THEN IT = IT + SA(1)
5590  IF T = > (DLY + SD(2)) THEN  RETURN
5600  IF T = > DLY THEN IT = IT + SA(2)
5620  RETURN
```

```
5700   REM    -> NEW VOLTAGE <-
5710 DV = IT * DT
5720 V = V - DV
5730 MV =  - V - 90
5740   RETURN
5750 :
5760 :
6000   REM -->PLOT AXES AND LABELS<--
6010   HGR : HOME
6020   HPLOT 25,151 TO 275,151
6030   FOR I = 0 TO 10
6040   HPLOT 25 + I * 25,152 TO 25 + I * 25,154
6050   NEXT I
6060   HPLOT 20,0 TO 20,86
6070   FOR I = 0 TO 13
6080   HPLOT 17,I * 6.67 TO 19,I * 6.67
6090   NEXT I
6100   HPLOT 15,20 TO 275,20
6110   HOME : VTAB 21
6120   HTAB 4: PRINT "0";
6130   HTAB 22: PRINT "5";
6140   HTAB 39: PRINT "10";
6150 :
6155   REM  DISPLAY STIMULUS PARAMETERS AT BOTTOM OF SCREEN
6160   VTAB 24: HTAB 1
6170   PRINT "#1=";SD(1);" @ ";SA(1);
6180   HTAB 17: PRINT "DELAY=";DL;
6190   HTAB 29
6200   PRINT "#2=";SD(2);" @ ";SA(2);
6205 :
6210   REM  PLOT INITIAL STEADY-STATE VALUES
6220   FOR X = 21 TO 24
6230   HPLOT X,20 - (MV / 1.5)
6240   HPLOT X,110
6250   HPLOT X,150 - 1.5 * GK
6260   HPLOT X,150 - 1.5 * GN
6270   NEXT X
6280   RETURN
6290 :
```

Chapter 13


CARDIAC ACTION POTENTIALS


Studies of the electrophysiology of the myocardium are
motivated by both clinical and theoretical considerations. The
factors determining the flow of transmembrane currents in the
heart are of practical interest because of their role in
fibrillation and in producing the electrocardiogram at the body
surface. The technical difficulties which have been overcome in
order to make voltage-clamp measurements on this tissue attest
to the depths of human intellectual curiousity and
determination. Computer simulation is used widely for
predicting the body surface potentials during the spread of
myocardial excitation and for quantitative evaluations of
postulated components of the membrane currents.

The success of the Hodgkin and Huxley model for
excitation in the squid axon prompted attempts to modify this
model for Purkinje fibers (Noble, 1962) for which there were
preliminary voltage-clamp observations. As the experimental
evidence has accummulated the models have grown in complexity.
The reader is referred to the reviews by Trautwein (1973), Mc
Allister, et al (1975), Reuter (1979), and Vassalle (1979). This
chapter is limited to a reconstruction of the action potential
of ventricular myocardial fibers as presented by Beeler and
Reuter (1977). This is chosen because of its simplicity as
compared to other published models. The teaching benefits from
the simulation presented are limited to plots of the kinetics of

James E. Randall, Microcomputers and Physiological Simulation

the hypothesized membrane currents in response to a rapid depolarization of the membrane. The model is sufficiently flexible so that knowledgeable cardiac electrophysiologists can demonstrate some features of cardiac arrhythmias and the actions of certain pharmacological agents (Cranefield and Wit, 1979).

The complexity of cardiac excitation imposes greater computational demands for simulation of the properties of this tissue than for the nerve axon. The time course of the cardiac process is slower, there are more components to the currents, and the formulations are more involved than in the axon models. In the Beeler and Reuter model for ventricular tissue there are four individual ionic currents considered while other models have postulated as many as eight. The initial excitatory event involves a fast inward current carried by sodium and having properties similar to the kinetics of this ion in the axon. There is a secondardy inward current, often called "slow inward", which is attributed to calcium and other ions. For brevity in program and graph labels this is referred to as calcium current.

A third component is an outward current, carried by potassium, which exhibits rectification properties and which depends upon potential but not upon time. The final component considered is a time- and voltage-dependent outward current carried mainly by potassium. The kinetics of the last three currents determine the time course of the plateau and repolarization phases of the action potential. The changes of the time-dependent conductances are governed by the products of dimensionless parameters which follow first-order kinetics with rate constants set by the membrane potential as in the Hodgkin and Huxley model.

The organization of this chapter is similar to that of the previous one. The computed variables are defined and used in BASIC equations for the functional relationships. Hodgkin-Huxey-type rate constants are evaluated for the existing membrane potential. These are used to update dimensionless "gating variables" which follow first-order differential equations. The four currents are evaluated and used to determine the net charge transferred during the integration interval. This provides a new membrane potential which is used in the next iteration.

The integration technique is the Euler method but alternative methods are described for improving accuracy and increasing speed. Except for graphic displays the programs should run on any microcomputer using BASIC. Tabular solutions are helpful for showing the absolute values of membrane currents, such as those which balance one another during the prolonged plateau. Because of the long duration of the action potential in cardiac tissue graphic solutions are more

effective.    Two different time scales are required in order to
see the  initial  rapid  inward  sodium  current  and  the  slow
repolarization  which  is completed several hundred milliseconds
later.   The Appendix contains the listing for a graphic solution
on the Apple II.

---

Table 13.1

An overview of the steps  in  the  simulation  of  the
ventricular  action potential.  The first section sets
up  the  parameters  and  determines  the  inititial
conditions.    The iteration loop provides for several
computations per output display according to the value
of CP set by the operator.

```
100 REM   -- BEELER-REUTER MODEL FOR VENTRICLE --
200 GOSUB 2000                    (Get parameters
300 GOSUB 3000                    (Rate constants
400 GOSUB 3200                    (Set variables
500 GOSUB 3700                    (Currents
600 GOSUB 6000                    (Plot axes,values
700 VM=V0                         (Initial potential
800 :
900 REM  LOOPS HERE FOR EACH OUTPUT <---------------
1000 GOSUB 4000                   (Output display
1100 FOR I= 1 TO CP               (CP=computes/output
1200     GOSUB 3000               (Set rate constants
1300     GOSUB 5000               (Update variables
1500     GOSUB 3700               (Update currents
1600     T=T+DT:VM=VM-IT*DT       (Update T & VM
1700     NEXT I                   (Ready to Output?
1800 GOTO 900                     (Repeat loop  ----->
```

---

FORMULATION IN BASIC

     The  program presented here consists of BASIC statements
which implement the relationships given in Table I of the/ paper
by  Beeler  and  Reuter  (1977).    Table 13.1 gives the general
layout of the simulation of their model as a series  of  modular
subroutine  calls  which  perform  specialized  functions.   The
subroutine  at  line  2000  asks  for  (or sets)  the  stimulus
parameters, the initial membrane potential, the initial internal
concentration of calcium, the integration increment DT, and  the
number of computations per output display.    The  subroutine

starting at line 3000 sets the steady-state rate constants according to the initial membrane potential while that at line 3200 sets the initial values of the dimensionless variables. These are followed by routines which set the initial values of dimenionless variables and which plot graphic axes if they are needed.

The iteration process consists of two imbedded loops. Lines 1000 through 1800 in Table 13.1 are executed for each output display until the process is terminated within the output subroutine, as at the end of a graphic display. The variable CP has been initialized previously to indicate how many times the membrane variables are to be updated between each output display. The inner loop, consisting of lines 1200-1600, sets the rate constants, calculates the currents, and then updates the membrane potential accordingly in line 1600.

Table 13.2 lists the variables used in the simulations of this chapter along with their steady-state values for a resting membrane potential of -84 mv, the value used by Beeler and Reuter. The symbols corrrespond to the variables used in their paper within the two-letter limitations of Microsoft BASIC version 4.0.

The rate constants in Table 13.2 are denoted by the letters A and B, corresponding to the greek letters alpha and beta used in the literature. The initial Na+ entry has kinetics determined by the product of the three dimensionless variables M, H, and J. The secondary current has an activation variable D and an inactivation variable F. Potassium permeability is modified by the activation factor, identified as X1 to distinguish it from the abscissa of a graph. The Beeler and Reuter model considers only four membrane currents, as mentioned above. IK is the voltage-dependent K+ current. IX is the voltage- and time- dependent K+ current. INA is the first inward component arising from Na+. IS is the secondary inward current containing Ca++. IT is the total current, including any externally applied stimulus. The convention used is that entry of positively charged ions is considered an inward current with a negative sign.

In considering the entry of Ca++ the model includes a reversal potential, ES, for this ion but its value changes as calcium enters the cell. CA is the initial value of intracellular calcium concentration, taken as $3*10^-7$ moles/l. Voltages throughout this model are electric potential differences with inside minus outside convention, denoted as VM. The symbol V0 is used for the value of the membrane potential at the beginning of the first iteration interval.

Table 13.2

Symbols and steady-state values of the variables used
in the BASIC simulation of the Beeler-Reuter model for
ventricular   action   potential.     The    potential
differences are inside minus outside.    The  entry  of
positive  ions  is considered as inward current with a
negative sign.  References  to  calcium  currents  and
rate  constants  apply  to  the  slow secondary inward
current.

| SYMBOL | VARIABLE | STEADY-STATE VALUE |
|---|---|---|
| | Rate constants | |
| AM | Alpha-M,Na+ off-on | 0.903  /msec |
| BM | Beta-M, Na+  on-off | 80.6        " |
| AH | Alpha-H,Na+  off-on | 0.822       " |
| BH | Beta-H, Na+  on-off | 0.010       " |
| AJ | Alpha-J,Na+  off-on | 0.060       " |
| BJ | Beta-J, Na+  on-off | 0.002       " |
| AD | Alpha-D,Ca++ off-on | 0.0004      " |
| BD | Beta-D, Ca++ on-off | 0.123       " |
| AF | Alpha-F,Ca++ off-on | 0.019       " |
| BF | Beta-F, Ca++ on-off | 3.5 E-7 /msec |
| AX | Alpha-X,K+   off-on | 2.5 E-5     " |
| BX | Beta-X, K+   on-off | 0.004       " |
| | Dimensionless variables | |
| M | Na+  activation | 0.011 |
| H | Na+  inactivation | 0.987 |
| J | Na+  inacativation | 0.975 |
| D | Ca++ activation | 0.003 |
| F | Ca++ inactivation | 1.000 |
| X1 | K+   activation | 0.006 |
| | Currents | |
| IK | V-depend. K+ | 0.472 µamp/sq cm |
| IX | T-depend. K+ | -0.009     " |
| INA | T-depend. Na+ | -0.404     " |
| IS | Slow (Ca++) | -0.055     " |
| IT | Total | 0.00      " |
| CA | Intracell Ca++ | 3.0 E-7 mole/l |
| | Voltages | |
| VM | inside-outside | -84.5 mv |
| V0 | at T=0 | |
| ES | Ca reversal | 113.  mv |

INITIAL CONDITIONS

    The initialization steps, given in lines 200-700 of
Table 13.1, are very similar to those in the previous chapter.
The major differences arise from what parameters are used and
the greater number of factors considered in setting the
steady-state cardiac conductances and currents. In the
illustrations in this chapter only a step change in membrane
potential is considered as the stimulus but there could be more
parameters involved as was done for the axon. For generality
the integration interval DT could be set by the operator as
could the number of computations between output displays. For
student use it is preferable to have these options fixed
according to a previous plan so that time is not wasted on less
rewarding combinations. The key steps for setting the
parameters as they are used in this chapter are

```
2000 REM  -- SET PARAMETERS --
2010 T = 0: CA = 3 E-7: VM = -84.5
2020 INPUT "DT = ? ";DT
2030 INPUT "COMPUTATIONS/PLOT = ";CP
2040 INPUT "STEP MV TO"; V0
2050 RETURN
```

---

### Table 13.3

The calculations of the four components of membrane
current in the Beeler-Reuter model. IX and IK are
outward currents of K+; INA and IS are inward
currents, primarily of Na+ and CA++, respectively.

```
3700 REM  -- SET CURRENTS --
3710 Z=EXP(.04*(VM+35))                    (Denominator
3720 IX=X1*(.8*(EXP(.04*(VM+77))-1)/Z)     (K f(V,T)
3730:
3740 INA=((4*M*M*M*H*J)+.003)*(VM-50)      (Initial Na+
3750:
3760 ES=-82.3-13.0287*LOG(CA)              (CA reversal
3770 IS=.09*D*F*(VM-ES)                     (Slow current
3780 :
3790 Z1=4*(EXP(0.04*(V+85))-1)
3800 Z2=EXP(.08*(VM+53))+EXP(.04*(VM+53))
3810 Z3=.2*(VM+23)/(1-EXP(-.04*(VM+23)))
3820 IK= 0.35*((Z1/Z2) + Z3)               (K f(V)
3830 :
3840 IT= IX + INA + IS + IK                (Total current
3850 RETURN
```

It is most instructive to consider the next three subroutines in reverse order, looking first at the calculation of the four membrane currents as given in Table 13.3. The voltage- and time-dependent outward current of K+ is calculated in two parts in lines 3710 and 3720. The factor X1 is the dimensionless variable which can have values between 0 and 1.0 and which responds to potential changes according to a first-order differential equation. The balance of the expression gives the K+ current under conditions in which X1 is at its maximum value (fully activated), as during the depolarized part of the action potential. The complexity of this equation arises from the fact that this current is a non-linear function of membrane potential VM and not a simple product of constant conductance and net electrochemical potential gradient. Instead, its magnitude tends to plateau at large values of VM.

The initial inward Na+ current, calculated in line 3740, does have a conductance factor and a driving force factor. The value 4 millimho/sq cm is the maximum possible conductance for full activation of this channel, the value 0.003 is a minimum background independent of activation kinetics. The M variable is an activation factor, used here to its third power. H and J are inactivation factors having different time constants. The value 50 is the reversal potential used for sodium. When VM=50 there is no driving force upon this ion.

The secondary current IS, calculated in line 3770, is based upon a driving force and a conductance. When the channel is fully activated the conductance is 0.09 millimho/sq cm. The time- and voltage-dependent characteristics of this membrane parameter are conveyed by the dimensionless variables D and F. Each of these respond to membrane voltage changes by first-order kinetics determined by rate constants. D is an activation factor which tends to increase with time after depolarization; F is an activation factor which starts high and falls with depolarization.

The driving force which determines the current IS is considered to involve both the electric potential VM and a concentration gradient for calcium, measured by its reversal potential ES. Since intracellular concentrations of this ion change significantly during an action potential the value of ES can not be considered a constant. Its calculation in line 3760 involves a natural log of CA, the present intracellular concentration. The membrane current of potassium which depends only upon VM is given by a complex nonlinear expression requiring four lines, 3790-3820. In line 3840 the total current is taken as the sum of the four which have just been computed. During a stimulus there is an additional component to the total current IT.

Table 13.4

Subroutines for evaluating rate constants and for
setting steady-state values of the dimensionless
variables.    Lines 3000-3150 use the empirical
relationships given in the Beeler and Reuter model for
the instantaneous values of the rate constants at
existing membrane potential VM.  Lines 3200-3270 use
these rate constants to set the steady-state values of
the six parameters which determine the time-dependent
changes of the membrane conductances.

```
3000 REM -- SET RATE CONSTANTS FOR MEMBRANE POTENTIAL --
3010 AM=(-1*(VM+47))/(EXP(-.1*(VM+47))-1)
3020 BM=(40*EXP(-.056*(VM+72)))
3030 AH=(.126*EXP(-.25*(VM+77)))
3040 BH=(1.7)/(EXP(-.082*(VM+22.5))+1)
3050 AJ=(.055*EXP(-.25*(VM+78)))/(EXP(-.2*(VM+78))+1)
3060 BJ=(.3)/(EXP(-.1*(VM+32))+1)
3070 :
3080 AD=(.095*EXP(-.01*(VM-5)))/(EXP(-.072*(VM-5))+1)
3090 BD=(.07*EXP(-.017*(VM+44)))/(EXP(.05*(VM+44))+1)
3100 AF=(.012*EXP(-.008*(VM+28)))/(EXP(.15*(VM+28))+1)
3110 BF=(.0065*EXP(-.02*(VM+30)))/(EXP(-.2*(VM+30))+1)
3120:
3130 AX=(.0005*EXP(.083*(VM+50)))/(EXP(.057*(VM+50))+1)
3140 BX=(.0013*EXP(-.06*(VM+20)))/(EXP(-.04*(VM+20))+1)
3150 RETURN
3160:
3170:
3200 REM  -- STEADY-STATE DIMENSIONLESS VARIABLES --
3210 M = AM / (AM+BM)
3220 H = AH / (AH+BH)
3230 J = AJ / (AJ+BJ)
3240 D = AD / (AD+BD)
3250 F = AF / (AF+BF)
3260 X1= AX / (AX+BX)
3270 RETURN
3280 :
```

    The time-dependent currents calculated in Table 13.3
require that the six dimensionless gating parameters, X1, M,  H,
J,  D,  and  F  each  be  evaluated using their respective rate
constants as determined by the initial steady-state membrane
potential.   Table 13.4 contains the subroutine starting at line
3200 which sets these parameters after the subroutine at line
3000 has evaluated the rate constants.

THE ITERATION LOOP

        Starting from the initial steady-state currents, lines 1200 through 1500 in Table 13.1 call in subroutines which determine the total current at the end of an integration interval. In line 1600 the net charge transferred (IT*DT) is used with a membrane capacity of 1 uF/sq cm to update the membrane potential for the next iteration. Line 1000 calls a subroutine starting at line 4000 which displays the desired computed variables, either in a tabular form or as a graphic function of time. The discussion of the alternatives for displaying the solutions is delayed until later in this chapter.

---

Table 13.5

Subroutine which calculates new values of the time-dependent activation and inactivation factors using an Euler approximation to the defining first-order differential equations. Line 5020 calculates the new cellular concentration of calcium.


```
5000 REM -- UPDATE TIME-DEPENDENT VARIABLES --
5010:
5020 CA = CA + DT * ((-1E-7*IS)+.07*((1E-7)-CA))
5030:
5040 M = M + DT * (AM*(1-M) - BM*M)
5050 H = H + DT * (AH*(1-H) - BH*H)
5060 J = J + DT * (AJ*(1-J) - BJ*J)
5070 D = D + DT * (AD*(1-D) - BD*D)
5070 F = F + DT * (AF*(1-F) - BF*F)
5080 X1 = X1 + DT * (AX*(1-X1) - BX*X1)
5090:
5100 RETURN
```

---

        Line 1200 calls the same subroutine at line 3000 (Table 13.4) to evaluate the alpha's and beta's for the current value of VM since these rate constants are not functions of time. However, it is necessary to have a subroutine to update the dimensionless variables according to an approximation for their defining first-order differential equations as in Table 13.5. This uses simple Euler integration which assumes constant changes of these variables over the integration interval. Later discussion indicates that this is unacceptably slow and so offers an alternative methods. The Euler routine is used here for the purpose of clarity and to follow the pattern of the previous chapter.

In addition to these conductance parameters it is
necessary to consider the change in intracellular calcium
concentration which occurs between the times T and T+DT. The
model for this step, given in line 5020, includes an
accumulation rate proportional to the slow inward current IS and
an elimination rate related to the cellular concentration CA.

---

| COMPUTED RESPONSES |
| --- |

Beeler and Reuter found that their four-current model
accounts for many of the experimental observations which have
been reported for the ventricular myocardium. However,
inadequate information is available concerning the kinetics
important in propagation, the intracellular ionic
concentrations, and the electrogenic pumping mechanisms. In
addition, the model describes the electrophysiology of
ventricular tissue which is much different from that of nodal
pacemakers and of the Purkinje system. Nevertheless, the fact
that the model contains only four components to the membrane
current makes it practical for solutions on microcomputers in
BASIC. These simulations can be used to introduce beginning
students to the complexity of action potentials from all parts
of the heart. They highlight the distinction between the "fast"
and the "slow" components of the inward current and provide
background for the topical subject of "slow responses."

The simulations presented in this section are done on
the Apple II microcomputer using the BASIC routines given in the
first section. However, the Euler integration in Table 13.5 is
replaced by a more efficient scheme which is described later in
this chapter. The solutions can be obtained in tabular form on
any computer which uses BASIC with an appropriate output
subroutine at line 4000. The integration intervals for the
examples in this section are reduced to a size that does not
influence the accuracy of the solution. The slowness of
simulations in BASIC is tolerable for lecture demonstrations but
machine-language numerical processor routines should be used
when students are expected to do several exercises on an
individual basis. The topic of accuracy and speed is also
considered in the next section.

THE STANDARD RESPONSE

Figure 13.1 shows the potential and current responses to
a step change in membrane potential from −84 to −55 mv as
computed by the Beeler and Reuter model. In order to improve
temporal and amplitude resolution these are presented in four
separate CRT displays. Later figures combine this information

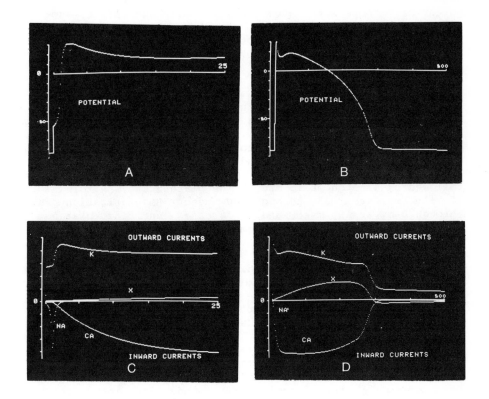

Figure 13.1.  Computed  membrane potential and current responses
    to a step change in membrane  potential  according  to  the
    model  of  Beeler  and  Reuter  for  ventricular myocardial
    fibers.  A) and B) contain membrane potential on  0-25  and
    0-500  msec  scales.  C) and D) show the corresponding four
    membrane  currents  with  depolarizing   currents   plotted
    downward.  The two inward currents are the fast Na+ and the
    slow secondary one labeled CA.  The outward currents,  both
    attributed  to potassium, are the time independent K, and a
    voltage- and time-dependent X.  The ordinate scale for  the
    Na current is in steps of 40 μamps/sq cm while that for the
    other three ions is in steps of 1 unit.  In all cases there
    are 250 points on the abscissa.  These are photographs from
    the  Apple  II  high-resolution   graphics  display   with
    lettering by user-defined vectors.

into  a single display to be viewed by student groups.  The time
scale of 0-25 msec, in 13.1A and 13.1C, is necessary to see  the
fast  inward  current of sodium and the rate of rise of membrane
potential.  Those with 0-500 msec, in 13.1B and  13.1D,  do  not
reveal  the  sodium current but show the full time course of the
repolarization phase.  The  bottom  two  panels  emphasize  the
direction  of  the  currents  by  having  outward (repolarizing)
currents plotted up and inward (depolarizing)  currents  plotted
down.

      Figure 13.1B, showing the complete time  course  of  the
action  potential,  is  comparable  to  Figure 4 in the paper by
Beeler and Reuter.  The  first  two  points  on  the  curve  are
connected  by  continuous  vectors  to highlight the step change
from  resting  potential  and  the  rapid  regenerative
depolarization.   The  peak of the spike, just below +30 mv, is
followed by a notch at 15 msec.  The plateau stays within  1  mv
of  +16  mv  from  35 through 80 msec.  Repolarization passes
through 0 mv at 155 msec and  progresses  until  a  plateau  is
reached  near  the  resting  membrane potential at 300 msec.  In
Figure 13.1A it can be seen that the maximum rate of  change  of
potential  is  about  12 mv within 0.1 msec, the temporal
resolution on this display.  This corresponds to a value of  120
v/sec.

      In the figure the initial inward  current,  carried  by
Na+,  has a scale 1/40th that used for the other three currents.
For Na+ each vertical interval is  40  µamp/sq  cm.   This  ion
reaches  its  peak value of -145 units at about 1 msec after the
initial step depolarization.  The behavior of this component  is
very similar to that for the sodium current in the axon since it
is  blocked  by  tetrodotoxin  (TTX)  and  is  influenced  by
extracellular  concentrations  of  sodium.  The kinetics of the
inactivation of this current  are  influenced  markedly  by  the
initial  degree  of  membrane  polarization,  a  topic  to  be
considered later.

      The  other currents in the figure are plotted with each
tic on the ordinate representing 1 µamp/sq cm.   The  secondary
inward  current labeled CA  in  the  figures,  rises  toward a
sustained peak value of -4 units.  Its time course  is  dictated
by  activation  and  inactivation factors which are voltage- and
time-dependent so  that  the  current  changes  lag  behind  the
voltage  changes.   A  major  component  of  this  current  is
considered  to  be  calcium,  but  other  ions  are  undoubtedly
involved  under  natural  and experimental conditions.  The slow
inward current is of topical interest because of its role in the
"slow  response",  described  later,  and  because  the  calcium
component is  a  link  between  excitation  and  contraction  in
cardiac muscle.   It  is  commonly thought that adrenergic and
cholinergic transmitters have a strong effect on this component.
As the action potential progresses the  falling  value  of  this

current is explained by the kinetics of its inactivation factor, denoted by F in the computer program. This parameter has a time constant measured in hundreds of millseconds when the intracellular potential is positive.

The two outward currents are considered in the model to be carried primarily by potassium. The one labeled K in the figures (IK in the computer programs) is a non-linear function of membrane potential which changes instantaneously. Thus in the simulations it will follow the changes in potentials without time delays, though not in a proportionate manner. This outward current acts to moderate the potential changes which occur as a result of the two inward currents and so contributes to the plateau phase of the action potential.

Because of its time-dependent nature the current labeled X, also carried by potassium, lags behind the membrane potential. It reaches a peak value of 1.2 units at 200 msec when it makes its contribution to the net outward current responsible for repolarization. Note that it has a net inward value at voltages more negative than -77 mv.

The sum of the four described currents at each time increment determine the charge which is transferred across the membrane and thus the change in membrane potential. When the net current is inward, as with Na+ activation during the first 3 msec, the membrane is depolarized. When the total current is small there is no change in potential, as during the plateau. When the total currents flowing inward become less than those outward repolarization occurs. The notch at the peak of the action potential is explained in the Beeler-Reuter model by the balance between the rising inward current and the steady K+ current outward. The Purkinje fiber model of McAllister et al (1975) required a choride current to produce such a notch. In the present model the repolarization process depends upon the deactivation of the secondary inward current so that it becomes less than the sum of the two outward K+ currents. In the final plateau which occurs after 300 msec the total membrane current is small. Figure 13.1D may appear to contradict this, but it must be recalled that the Na+ current, which has a value of -0.4 units at this time, is plotted to 1/40th the scale of the other three currents.


SODIUM CURRENT AND RATE OF DEPOLARIZATION

During the normal depolarization process the total membrane current is completely dominated by the rapid influx of sodium. Thus the rate of change of the rising phase of the action potential is often taken as a measure of the sodium current and its kinetics. This topic is of practical interest because the rate of change of membrane potential is a

significant factor in setting the velocity of propagation in
excitable tissue, and even determines whether a given segment is
excited.    It  is possible that some pharmacological agents may
exert their influences upon conduction by altering the entry  of
sodium  and  thus  the  rate  of  change  of  potential.    Both
experimental and modeling studies show that the rate of rise  of
potential   is    diminished   when    the    process   starts  from
steady-state potentials which are depolarized relative to normal
values.    The  term membrane "responsiveness" is used widely to
refer to the idea that maximum rate of change of potential is   a
function of the membrane potential at which it is elicited.

     The simulations in Figures 13.2 and 13.3 illustrate   how
the   steady-state   potentials  determine   the   Na+   current   and
voltage rise in the Beeler-Reuter model.   These    authors   found
the   responsiveness  to  be  at a maximum for initial potentials
more negative than -80 mv and diminished to very low   values   at
potentials more positive than -60 mv.  In these two figures, and
in those in the remainder of the chapter, the inward and outward
currents  are   all plotted upward.  The ordinate tic corresponds
to 100 µamps/sq cm for the Na+ current and to 5 µamps/sq cm   for
the   others.   The Na+ tracing generally can be identified by its
short duration, about 2 msec.     The   K+  tracing  follows   the
membrane   potential   without   a   time   delay.    The slow inward
current (CA) is represented by a broken line.   Changes   in   the
time-dependent  K+  tracing  lag  behind  those  of the membrane
potential.    Color   graphics   can   be   used   effectively   to
distinguish between these overlapping tracings.

Fig. 13.2.    Computed  membrane
currents        and        potential
responses   for   a   step  change
depolarization during a 10 msec
sweep.   Both inward and outward
currents   are   plotted . upward.
Sodium current reaches   a   peak
value  of  -145 µamps/sq cm at 1
msec, and sets the maximum rate
of   depolarization.    The  other
three currents are on   a   scale
of   0-5  µamps/sq  cm. The slow
inward currrent is   represented
with a broken line.

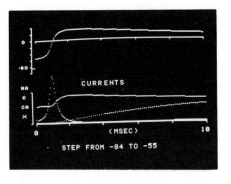

     Figure 13.2 shows the response starting from an   initial
membrane  potential  of  -84 mv, a value at which the activation
(D) and inactivation (F) dimensionless  variables  respond  to
provide  the  large  peak  in  sodium  current at 1 msec. This
current determines the rate of rise of the potential in the  top
tracing  of  the  figure.     This  is to be contrasted with the

situation in Figure 13.3 where the initial potential is at -72.5
mv, a value at which the time constant of the activation
variable D is increased, accounting for the slower rise in
sodium response which now peaks after 2 msec. The reduced Na+
current results in a slower rate of rise of membrane potential
and a reduced amplitude.

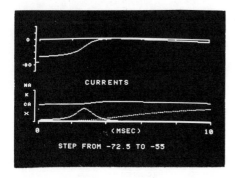

Fig. 13.3. The same responses
as in Fig. 13.2 expect that
the membrane starts from an
intitial potential of -72.5
mv. Under this condition the
sodium activation time
constant is significantly
prolonged so that the rise in
fast inward current is delayed
and reduced.

Beeler and Reuter found that the properties of the
membrane responsiveness following steady-state conditions can be
explained by the product of the two Na+ dimensionless variables
D and F. On the other hand, the rate of change of potential
starting from the same voltages on the repolarization phase of
the action potential indicates that additional factors are
involved in membrane responsiveness under these conditions.


THE SLOW RESPONSE

Slow action potentials can be generated from membranes
in which the sodium entry is absent either because of low
extracellular concentration or because of inactivation by
membrane depolarization as described above. These "slow
responses" are "calcium action potentials" because they depend
upon the regenerative entry of the secondary inward current. It
has been suggested by Cranefield (1975) that certain arrhythmias
may result from a more positive resting membrane potential which
deactivates the sodium entry and leaves only a slow response.

As has been found for certain experimental conditions
the present simulation provides oscillatory behavior for
constant depolarizing current without the intervention of
sodium. Figure 13.4 presents a 2.5 sec simulation in which the
sodium current is set to zero and the total membrane current
contains a constant depolarizing stimulus of 2.5 µamps/sq cm.
In this run the build up of intracellular positive charge starts
the entry of the secondary current which is plotted as a broken
line. The depolarization starts the lagged outward K+ current
and inactivates the slow inward current starting repolarization.

Fig. 13.4. An oscillatory
response produced by a constant
depolarizing stimulus of 2.5
µamps/sq cm. The fact that
sodium current is not included
in this modification of the
model suggests that pacemaker
activity could be sustained
in the absence of sodium
activation. The total membrane
current contains the 2.5 units
of stimulus not shown on the
graphs of individual currents.

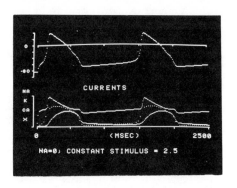

During the period from 0.7 to 1.3 sec the constant stimulus
gradually depolarizes the membrane again until threshold is
reached to start the regenerative slow response at 1.5 seconds.
The time course of the rate of rise of potential is dependent
upon the kinetics of the secondary current activation and
deactivation processes, both of which are at least an order of
magnitude slower than those for sodium.

        In their paper Beeler and Reuter compared simulations
for steady depolarizing current stimuli with and without the
sodium current. The only contribution of the sodium current was
to speed up the first depolarization. Thereafter the subsequent
action potentials were undistinguishable except for the lag of
the sodium-free train. This was because the repolarization
process never returned the membrane to a potential sufficiently
negative to reactivate the sodium process in the version which
included that ion. With only the background leakage of sodium
the behavior is similar to that for no sodium.

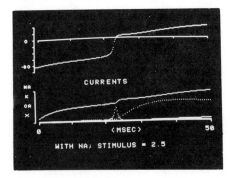

Fig. 13.5. The responses to
constant depolarizing currents
when sodium current is
included. At the threshold
for Na+ activation the entry
of this ion rapidly
depolarizes the membrane,
acting to advance the overall
process.

Figure 13.5 illustrates how the presence of sodium acts to modify the simulation given in the previous figure for a constant stimulus. In the case with sodium, for the first 20 msec there is a ramp of depolarization produced by the net entry of stimulating current over the exit of the voltage-dependent K+ current. When the voltage reaches the threshold for the Na+ activation there is a small pulse of sodium entry which rapidly depolarizes the membrane to a higher value. This rapid advancement in membrane potential is the role that the sodium plays in the oscillatory response. Subsequently the potential never becomes negative enough to allow the sodium process to be activated again.

A final simulation illustrates the regenerative entry of the slow current under circumstances in which the fast current is inactivated. In Figure 13.6 the initial membrane potential is at -67.5 mv, a value chosen to suppress sodium activation. When the potential is stepped to -5 mv the activation of the slow current allows positive ions to enter, even exceeding the loss of K+. At that point the potential begins to rise becoming even positive. This condition persists until the slow outward current, X, is activated at about 75 msec and then repolarization begins.

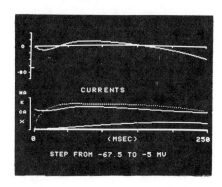

Fig. 13.6. Stepping the membrane from a voltage of -67.5 to -5 mv does not involve a sodium current. When the secondary inward current, the dotted line in the display, exceeds the outward K+ current the membrane begins to further depolarize beyond that of the original disturbance.

## OUTPUT DISPLAY AND COMPUTATION METHODS

The computation loop which updates activation parameters, currents, and membrane voltage takes 1.85 seconds per iteration when done in Applesoft BASIC. At this rate the total time to compute and display a graph of 250 points takes almost 8 minutes, too long for students to go through a set of self-teaching exercises. The author has reduced this time to 30 seconds by using a numerical processor chip and machine language programming for the 8080 microprocessor in an S-100 bus computer. The BASIC programs given in this chapter can be used

effectively in computers with graphics features for lecture
demonstrations or for individuals who are particularly motivated
to learn the properties of the Beeler-Reuter model. The purpose
of this section is to offer comments about methods which improve
the speed of these computations for teaching simulations.


GRAPHIC DISPLAYS

The figures in this chapter are CRT photographs from the
Apple II microcomputer. Following the plan given in Table 13.1,
a subroutine is placed starting at line 6000 which uses the
vector commands to draw the axes and tics. The high-resolution
graphics mode of Applesoft BASIC does not support intermixed
text and graphs so the user must supply labels by separate
software. Since only a few characters are needed in these
displays the expedient thing is to define those needed as a
sequence of vectors contained in a subroutine. For Figures 13.2
through 13.6 the HGR mode provides four lines of text at the
bottom of the screen. These contain the labels for the time
axis and a message related to the disturbance which initiates
the displayed response. Thus a single program provides
considerable flexibility in display format.

The subroutine at line 4000 displays the computed
variables using the Applesoft HPLOT X,Y command with an origin
in the upper left corner of the CRT screen. Each variable must
be scaled and provided with an offset to keep them within the
range on the screen. The main features include

```
4000 REM  -- APPLE GRAPHICS DISPLAY SUBROUTINE --
4010 X = 25 + 250 * (T/LX)                (Abcissa
4020 HPLOT X, 150 - ABS(INA/2)            (Sodium current
4030 HPLOT X, 150 - ABS(IX * 10)          (K+ f(V,T)
4040 HPLOT X, 150 - ABS(IK * 10)          (K+ f(T)
4050 IF X/3 - INT(X/3)<2/3 THEN GOTO 4070
4060 HPLOT X, 150 - ABS(IS * 10)          (2 of 3 slow
4070 IF X =<  275 THEN RETURN
4080 REM  COMES HERE AFTER 250 POINTS
4090 :
```

The variable LX in line 4010 is previously set to the value of T
for the last x-coordinate which is located at 275 on the screen.
The scaled currents are plotted above a baseline at a
y-coordinate of 150. Line 4050 skips plotting the slow current
every third value of X to give that tracing an identifiable
appearance. If a color monitor is available each current can be
displayed in a different color using the HCOLOR command of the
Apple computer. As soon as the x-coordinate reaches its last
value of 275 the subroutine no longer returns to the main
iteration loop but rather goes into some kind of a software halt
until a command is given to restart the simulation.

ACCURACY

        The   major   consideration   regarding   accuracy   of   the
simulation for this model involves the method of integrating the
first-order  differential  equations which describe the rates of
change of the dimensionless variables and the currents.   Beeler
and  Reuter  used  a  version of the Runge-Kutta algorithm which
uses five evaluations of the  derivatives  at  each  integration
step.   The  method allows adjusting the step size according to
the estimates of the error and according  to  the  fastest  time
constant  which is involved in the simulation. While suited for
research  computations  at  very  large  computer  centers  such
methods  are  not feasible for microcomputer simulations at this
time.

        The   program  in  Table  13.5  updates the time-dependent
variables using simple Euler integration.  The author finds that
this  method  requires integration step sizes of no greater than
0.01 msec in order to provide stable  solutions  of  the  sodium
activation  variable  M  which  has  a very short time constant.
Using this method requires 200 iterations during the duration of
the  Na+ activation process, an unreasonable amount to add on to
the  time  required  to  compute  the  balance  of  the  action
potential.  The author uses a modified Euler method described by
Moore  and  Ramon  (1974)  and  by  Rush  and  Larsen  (1978)  in
references  cited  in  Chapter  12.   This  algorithm  provides
essentially the same Na+ current curve at integration  intervals
of  either  0.01 or 0.1 msec so this is used as a criterion that
the method provides reasonable accuracy.   In  addition,  with
DT=0.1  msec  during  the  Na+  activation  process  the overall
displays of currents and  potentials  appear  to  be  reasonable
approximations  of  the solutions of Beeler and Reuter, at least
for teaching applications with microcomputers.

        The   essence  of  the finite integration, which Dr. John
Moore called a modified  Euler  method,  is that it  assumes  that
the  dimensionless  variables  change  exponentially  during the
integration interval.  Consider the Na+ activation variable M as
an  example.   It starts from its value at the beginning of the
integration interval and  changes  exponentially  toward  a  new
steady-state value determined by the rate constants AM and BM as
set by the membrane potential at  the  end  of  the  integration
interval.   The time constant TM of this change is determined by
the quantity TM = 1/(AM+BM).  However, this time constant may be
much  longer than the integration interval so that the change of
M during DT is calculated using the factor EXP(-DT/DM).   Table
13.6  presents  a  replacement  for  the  Euler steps used in Table
13.5.

        In   this   subroutine line 5020 updates the intracellular
calcium concentration as before.  The balance of the routine  is
concerned with updating the variables M, H, J, D, F, and X1 from

their values at the beginning of the last DT interval to those
to be used for the next one. Upon entering the subroutine the
respective rate constants, e.g., AM and BM, have been set to the
values determined by the membrane potential at end of the last
interval.   The assumption is that during the last interval the
variables will start an exponential change toward a new
steady-state value, e.g., MS=AM/(AM+BM) with a time constant
TM=1/(AM+BM).   However, this final value is never reached
because after time DT there are new values of rate constants.
Line 5200 sets the two parameters according to the rate
constants AM and BM.  Line 5210 replaces the previous value of M
with a new one.  The quantity (MS-M) is the total change in M
over an infinite time.  The quantity EXP(-DT/TM) is the fraction
of that change realized within the time DT.  These are combined
to give the new value of M.  Similar operations are performed on
the other five dimensionless variables.

Table 13.6

The suggested alternative for the Euler integration
method of Table 13.5.  Rather than assuming a constant
change in the parameters this method assumes an
exponential change during the integration increment
DT.   The time constants and infinite-time values are
calculated from the rate constants.

```
5000 REM -- UPDATE TIME-DEPENDENT VARIABLES --
5010 :
5020 CA = CA + DT * ((-1E-7*IS)+.07*((1E-7)-CA))
5030 :
5200 MS = AM/(AM+BM): TM = 1/(AM+BM)
5210 M = MS - (MS-M) * EXP(-DT/TM)
5220 :
5230 HS = AH/(AH+BH): TH = 1/(AH+BH)
5240 H = HS - (HS-H) * EXP(-DT/TH)
5250 :
5260 JS = AJ/(AJ+BJ): TJ = 1/(AJ+BJ)
5270 J = JS - (JS-J) * EXP(-DT/TJ)
5280 :
5290 DS = AD/(AD+BD): TD = 1/(AD+BD)
5300 D = DS - (DS - D) * EXP(-DT/TD)
5310 :
5320 FS = AF/(AF+BF): TS = 1/(AF+BF)
5330 F = FS - (FS-F) * EXP(-DT/TS)
5340:
5350 XS = AX/(AX+BX): TX = 1/(AX+BX)
5360 X1 = XS - (XS-X1) * EXP(-DT/TX)
5370 RETURN
```

This method requires a time-consuming exponential that
is not in the Euler method, but its use appears to permit
shortening the integration interval to achieve a significant
gain in computation speed. This method is used in all of the
figures in this chapter and in each case the author has
satisfied himself that the responses were not significantly
improved by shortening the integration step size. In
simulations in which there is no sodium or after sodium
inactivation has occurred the integration step size can be
increased to 1 msec, or even larger, with no noticeable effect
upon the displayed solutions.


SPEED

The evaluation of the exponential functions and the
number of differential equations take considerable time for
simulation of the ventricular action potential in BASIC. The
1.85 seconds required for each iteration in Applesoft involves
0.9 sec for evaluating the rate constants because of the 19
exponentials involved. The updating of the activation
variables, involving 6 exponentials, takes 0.25 sec. The
calculation of new currents takes 0.55 sec because of the
exponentials in the non-linear expressions for IK and IX in
addition to the logarithm in the expression for the secondary
current. The graphics and other items contribute 0.15 sec.
Efforts for speed improvement using interpreter languages must
eliminate the need for evaluating the exponentials and adjust
the size of the integration step.

If the microcomputer has an extra 22K bytes for storage
of variables the 12 rate constants can be stored as subscripted
elements in arrays as described in the chapter on axon
excitation. If the rate constants are each evaluated in 1 mv
increments between -100 and +40 mv the routines which use them
should contain subscripts, such as AM(J) and BM(J), where
J=INT(VM)+101. Thus upon each iteration the time is spent in
looking for the appropriate value in the array, an operation
which is much quicker than evaluating the function.
Incorporating this feature reduces the iteration time from 1.85
to 1 sec without any apparent loss in accuracy. The 4.1 minutes
for computing and displaying 250 points is a significant
reduction from the alternative of 8 minutes.

There are problems associated with this mode of
operation. It takes time to put the 1,680 13-digit elements
into the array. Computation of the total set takes 2.5 minutes.
Calling the values from a file on disk also may take significant
time. Some kinds of errors wipe out the array area from memory.
A program which has adequate protection against errors and which
is to be rerun several times in succession will benefit from
this method of reducing simulation time.

The size of the integration step required for the sodium activation stages is unnecessarily small for the simulation which occurs after sodium inactivation. For DT=0.01 or 0.1 msec the peak sodium current inward is -145 units at 1 msec after the suprathreshold depolarization from -84 mv. The primary manifestation of this is the rate of rise of potential and the extent of the postive overshoot. For fidelity of the initial phase DT should be no greater than 0.1 msec but it can be increased to 1 msec after the sodium entry is completed.

For simulations which encompass 500 msec reasonable waveforms are achieved with DT=1 msec. This increment reduces the peak inward sodium to -50 units so that the initial spike is reduced somewhat, but the overall processes appear similar. Further increases in the step size are possible in the repolarization phase. Of course, such procedures must be used with caution for physiological realism but they can speed up program debugging time and display general trends when time must be minimized.

NUMERICAL PROCESSORS

Floating point hardware, such as the Am-9511 Arithmetic Processor Unit (APU) described in Chapter 4, is essential for student exercises which require several runs. The remarks at the end of the previous chapter (pages 191-194) are equally valid here. High-level languages which use the APU to replace software floating point computation routines will run about two to three times faster. A speed advantage of about ten times is gained if the computations and plotting can be done in machine language, but the programming efforts are tedious.

The recommended procedure for writing machine language versions is to first acquire a functioning BASIC program. Then, in the manner illustrated for the axon on page 194, replace each BASIC statement with an equivalent set of subroutine calls which utilize the Am-9511 for computation. The author has done this for the cardiac action potential model for an S-100 bus microcomputer which uses the 8080 microprocessor. Graphic responses at 250 increments of time are calculated and displayed within 30 seconds. BASIC is used to ask for the initial conditions and stimulus parameters.

REFERENCES

Beeler, G. W., and H. Reuter:    Reconstruction of the action
potential of ventricular myocardial fibres.    J. Physiol.
268:177-210 (1977).

Cranefield, P. F., and A. L. Wit: Cardiac Arrhythmias. Ann.
Rev. Physiol. 41:459-472 (1979).

Cranefield, P. F.:  The conduction of the cardiac impulse. Mount
Kisco, NY: Futura (1975).

Noble, D.:    A modification of  the Hodgkin-Huxley equations
applicable to Purkinje fibre action and  pace-maker  potentials.
J. Physiol. 160:317-352 (1962).

Reuter, H.:  Properties of two inward membrane currents  in  the
heart.  Ann. Rev. Physiol. 41:413-424 (1979).

Trautwein, W.: Membrane  currents  in  cardiac  muscle  fibers.
Physiol. Rev. 53:793-835 (1973).

Vassalle, M.:   Electrogenesis of  the  plateau  and  pacemaker
potential. Ann. Rev. Physiol. 41:425-440 (1979).

APPENDIX

    The  following  pages contain a listing of the essential
portions of the  Applesoft  BASIC  program  which  produces  the
simulations  used in Figures 13.2 through 13.6.  Omitted are the
vector plotting  routines  which  place  characters  within  the
graphics  area.   The subroutine at line 4000 has to be modified
to use this program on microcomputers  having  different  output
displays.   The remaining portions are compatible with Microsoft
BASIC which is popular for many microcomputers.

```
10   REM   APPLESOFT BASIC LISTING
15   REM    CARDIAC ACTION POTENTIAL AND CURRENTS
20   REM    MODEL OF REUTER AND BEELER
25   REM    J. PHYSIOL. 268:177-210 (1977)
97 :
98 :
99 :
100   REM  -- GET PARAMETERS, INITIALIZE STEADY STATE --
200   GOSUB 2000: REM     --GET PARAMETERS
300   GOSUB 3000: REM     --RATE CONSTANTS
400   GOSUB 3200: REM     --SET VARIABLES
500   GOSUB 3700: REM     --CURRENTS
600   GOSUB 6000: REM     --PLOT AXES, SS VALUES
700   VM = V0: REM        --INITIAL POTENTIAL
898 :
899 :
900 : REM    LOOPS HERE FOR EACH OUTPUT <-----------
1000   GOSUB 4000: REM       --DISPLAY OUTPUT
1100   FOR I = 1 TO CP
1200   :: GOSUB 3000: REM     --SET RATE CONSTANTS
1300   :: GOSUB 5000: REM     --UPDATE VARIABLES
1500   :: GOSUB 3700: REM     --UPDATE CURRENTS
1600   :::T = T + DT:VM = VM - IT * DT
1700   :: NEXT I
1800   GOTO 900: REM     --- REPEAT LOOP  ------->>
1997 :
1998 :
1999 :
2000   REM  -- SET PARAMETERS --
2005   TEXT : HOME :T = 0:CA = 3E - 7
2030   INPUT "DT = ?";DT
2040   INPUT "COMPUTE/PLOT = ";CP
2050   INPUT "MAX TIME ON CRT = ";LX
2060   INPUT "STEADY-STATE MV = ";VM
2070   INPUT "STEP MV TO ";V0
2080   INPUT "CONSTANT STIMULUS = ";ST
2090   RETURN
2997 :
2998 :
2999 :
3000   REM  -- SET RATE CONSTANTS FOR VM --
3010 Z = ( - 1 * (VM + 47))
3015 AM = Z / ( EXP ( - .1 * (VM + 47)) - 1)
3019 :
3020 BM = (40 *  EXP ( - .056 * (VM + 72)))
3025 :
3030 AH = (.126 *  EXP ( - .25 * (VM + 77)))
3035 :
3040 BH = 1.7 / ( EXP ( - .082 * (VM + 22)) + 1)
3049 :
3050 Z = (.055 *  EXP ( - .25 * (VM + 78)))
3055 AJ = Z / ( EXP ( - .2 * (VM + 78)) + 1)
```

```
3059  REM    CONTINUATION OF RATE CONSTANTS
3060  BJ = .3 / ( EXP ( - .1 * (VM + 32)) + 1)
3070  :
3080  Z = (.095 *  EXP ( - .01 * (VM - 5)))
3085  AD = Z / ( EXP ( - .072 * (VM - 5)) + 1)
3089  :
3090  Z = (.07 *  EXP ( - .017 * (VM + 44)))
3095  BD = Z / ( EXP (.05 * (VM + 44)) + 1)
3099  :
3100  Z = (.012 *  EXP ( - .008 * (VM + 28)))
3105  AF = Z / ( EXP (.15 * (VM + 28)) + 1)
3109  :
3110  Z = (.0065 *  EXP ( - .02 * (VM + 30)))
3115  BF = Z / ( EXP ( - .2 * (VM + 30)) + 1)
3120  :
3130  Z = (.0005 *  EXP (.083 * (VM + 50)))
3135  AX = Z / ( EXP (.057 * (VM + 50)) + 1)
3139  :
3140  Z = (.0013 *  EXP ( - .06 * (VM + 20)))
3145  BX = Z / ( EXP ( - .04 * (VM + 20)) + 1)
3149  :
3150  RETURN
3160  :
3170  :
3180  :
3200  REM  -- STEADY-STATE DIMENSIONLESS VARIABLES --
3210  M = AM / (AM + BM):H = AH / (AH + BH)
3230  J = AJ / (AJ + BJ):F = AF / (AF + BF)
3260  X1 = AX / (AX + BX)
3280  :
3285  :
3290  :
3700  REM  -- CALCULATE MEMBRANE              CURRENTS --
3710  Z =  EXP (.04 * (VM + 35))
3720  IX = X1 * (.8 * ( EXP (.04 * (VM + 77)) - 1) / Z)
3730  :
3740  INA = ((4 * M * M * M * H * J) + .003) * (VM - 50)
3750  :
3760  ES =  - 82.3 - 13.0287 *  LOG (CA)
3770  IS = .09 * D * F * (VM - ES)
3780  :
3790  Z1 = 4 * ( EXP (.04 * (VM + 85)) - 1)
3800  Z2 =  EXP (.08 * (VM + 53)) +  EXP (.04 * (VM + 53))
3810  Z3 = .2 * (VM + 23) / (1 -  EXP ( - .04 * (VM + 23)))
3820  IK = 0.35 * ((Z1 / Z2) + Z3)
3830  :
3840  IT = IX + INA + IS + IK + ST
3860  RETURN
```

```
4000   REM  -- OUTPUT DISPLAY ROUTINE --
4090 X = 25 + 250 * (T / LX): HPLOT X,20 - (VM / 2)
4110   HPLOT X,150 -  ABS (INA / 2)
4119   IF (X / 3) -  INT (X / 3) < 1 / 3 THEN  GOTO 4130
4120   HPLOT X,150 -  ABS (IS * 10)
4130   HPLOT X,150 -  ABS (IX * 10): HPLOT X,150 -  ABS (IK * 10)
4150   IF X =  < 275 THEN  RETURN
4200   GET A$
4210   GOTO 100
4220 :
4998 :
4999 :
5000   REM  -- UPDATE TIME-DEPENDENT VARIABLES --
5020 CA = CA + DT * (( - 1E - 7 * IS) + .07 * ((1E - 7) - CA))
5100 :
5200 MS = AM / (AM + BM):TM = 1 / (AM + BM)
5210 M = MS - (MS - M) *  EXP ( - DT / TM)
5220 :
5230 HS = AH / (AH + BH):TH = 1 / (AH + BH)
5240 H = HS - (HS - H) *  EXP ( - DT / TH)
5250 :
5260 JS = AJ / (AJ + BJ):TJ = 1 / (AJ + BJ)
5270 J = JS - (JS - J) *  EXP ( - DT / TJ)
5280 :
5290 DS = AD / (AD + BD):TD = 1 / (AD + BD)
5300 D = DS - (DS - D) *  EXP ( - DT / TD)
5310 :
5320 FS = AF / (AF + BF):TF = 1 / (AF + BF)
5330 F = FS - (FS - F) *  EXP ( - DT / TF)
5340 :
5350 XS = AX / (AX + BX):TX = 1 / (AX + BX)
5360 X1 = XS - (XS - X1) *  EXP ( - DT / TX)
5370   RETURN
5996 :
5997 :
5998 :
6000   REM  -- AXES AND INITIAL VALUES --
6005   HGR
6010   HPLOT 25,20 TO 275,20: HPLOT 19,0 TO 19,70
6020   FOR I = 0 TO 5
6030 : HPLOT 25 + I * 50,21 TO 25 + I * 50,22
6040 : HPLOT 25 + I * 50,151 TO 25 + I * 50,153: NEXT
6050   FOR I = 0 TO 7: HPLOT 17,I * 10 TO 18,I * 10: NEXT
6060   HPLOT 19,100 TO 19,150
6090   HPLOT 17,100 TO 18,100: HPLOT 17,150 TO 18,150
6110   HPLOT 25,150 TO 275,150
6120   VTAB 21: HTAB 4: PRINT "0";: HTAB 20: PRINT "(MSEC)";
6140   HTAB (41 -  LEN ( STR$ (LX))): PRINT  STR$ (LX)
6160   FOR X = 20 TO 24: HPLOT X,20 - (VM / 2): NEXT
6200   RETURN
```

Chapter 14

FORMATTING STUDENT EXERCISES

The theme of this book is the application of
microcomputers for mathematical simulation of physiological
processes, particularly for student self-study. The previous
chapters have focused upon the programming and expected
responses for several models with a few scattered references to
the interactive features which involve operator responses.
Regardless of how realistically the model may mimic a living
system it will have little teaching benefit if its performance
is obscured by the complexities of computer operation. Indeed,
one of the major advantages of microcomputers over the terminals
of time-shared macrocomputers is that the accessibility and
convenience of the inexpensive hardware should help overcome the
technical apprehension exhibited by many biology students. This
need will diminish as computer technology becomes commonplace in
secondary education but at the moment many students (and
faculty) view computer operation as beyond their capabilities.

This chapter summarizes some of the programming formats
and tricks which the author has used. All of these are obvious
once they are pointed out but the topic seems to be of
sufficient importance to warrant special attention.
Implementation will vary with the type of microcomputer and the
version of BASIC being used, but the material here is presented
in terms of the Apple II and Applesoft BASIC because of the
advantages of this system as described before. Many other
microcomputers can achieve the same results.

James E. Randall, Microcomputers and Physiological Simulation

---
TURNKEY SYSTEMS
---

It has been said that the first two minutes of  computer
operation   are   the   critical   ones   for converting novices into
permanent users of this hardware.  If attention must continually
be  focused  upon  the operating procedure at the expense of the
real objectives of the exercises the learning rewards may be  so
insignicant that the student will never return.  It is true that
with sufficient repetition anyone   can   relegate   the   secondary
procedures   to   spinal   reflexes, just as one learns to drive an
automobile, but this requires motivation of some form.   Turnkey
computer  systems, which start executing programs when the power
switch is turned on, are analogous  to   automatic   transmissions
which   help  beginning  drivers  enjoy  driving  without  being
burdened with learning the operation of the manual gear shift.

The   first   microcomputer models were miniature versions
of the large systems in that they had a panel  of  switches  and
lights with which an operator could exam memory locations, start
the programs at  arbitrary  locations,  and  debug  programs  by
executing  them  a  single command at a time.  These are popular
with technical hobbyists who enjoy the ability to interact  with
the  microprocessor  logic at the most basic level.  However the
simple task of starting a program  written  in  BASIC  on  these
machines  generally  requires the setting of several switches in
specific patterns and the issuing of commands involving  numbers
to  the  bases of 8 or of 16.  To broaden the market more recent
manufacturers have reduced the console to a typewriter  keyboard
with a few special purpose keys which are appropriately named.

As an example of an effective turnkey system, the  Apple
II  can  be  purchased with an Auto-start ROM (read-only-memory)
chip which executes a permanent program as soon as the power  is
turned  on.   This in turn initializes the disk operating system
(DOS) and calls in the first  program  on  the  diskette.   The
programmer  can  have  this  program do  anything  within  the
capabilities of any of the BASIC programs. It can give operating
instructions,  outline  the objectives of the teaching exercise,
or load and start another program from disk.

Figure  14.1  is  a  photograph of the CRT display which
appears about 5 seconds after the power  switch  is  turned  on.
This  is  the result of the first program on the disk so that it
is necessary that the disk be in place in its drive unit.  There
is  no reason that the disk can not be left in this location for
days at a time, secure and always ready to go when the power  is
turned  on.   This  particular  display  format, often called a
"menu", presents the different exercises on the disk identifying
them  by  number or letter.  The display stays there waiting for
the  student  to make a selection.  On a CRT with 24 lines there

is room for only nine or ten titles, but it is possible to have
one of these branch to second or third "pages" which exhibit
additional possibilities.

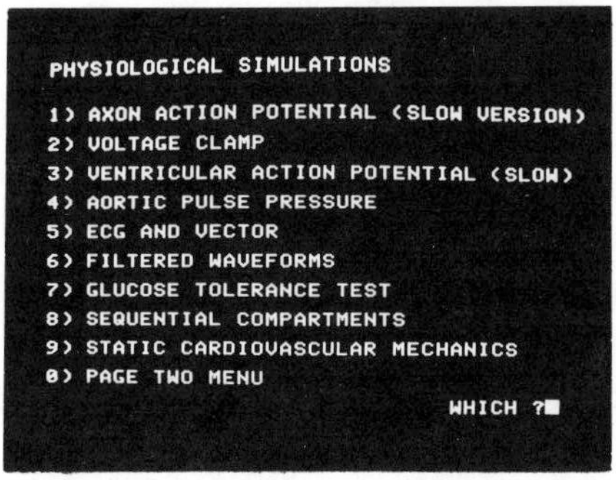

Fig. 14.1 The CRT upon turning
on a microcomputer with turnkey
capabilities.       The student
selects the exercise by number
and the corresponding program
is read in from disk. Thus no
technical skills are required
to start the simulations.

```
PHYSIOLOGICAL SIMULATIONS

1) AXON ACTION POTENTIAL (SLOW VERSION)
2) VOLTAGE CLAMP
3) VENTRICULAR ACTION POTENTIAL (SLOW)
4) AORTIC PULSE PRESSURE
5) ECG AND VECTOR
6) FILTERED WAVEFORMS
7) GLUCOSE TOLERANCE TEST
8) SEQUENTIAL COMPARTMENTS
9) STATIC CARDIOVASCULAR MECHANICS
0) PAGE TWO MENU
                              WHICH ?
```

The WHICH? question is followed by an INPUT statement
waiting for a selected number or letter. For many versions of
BASIC such an entry must be terminated by pressing the RETURN
key.   Since this termination may not be obvious to the
first-time user there is an advantage to using the GET A$
command which assigns the single alphanumerical character
pressed to the string variable A$ without waiting for a RETURN
termination. This sets the hesitant newcomer off into the
simulation immediately.   However the user who automatically
terminates every entry with a RETURN may find that he has
already answered the next inquiry prematurely.   Note that
superious entries outside the indicated range should be ignored
by the program.

Once the title has been selected an ON .... GOTO ...
statement branches the menu program to commands which load the
proper exercise from disk and start it.   This may take from five
to ten seconds or longer if there are machine-language routines
to be loaded also. This time should not be wasted.   After the
WHICH? question is answered the program should clear the screen
and reinforce the name of the chosen exercise, state its
objectives, and perhaps give credit to its source. This text
will stay on the screen while the program and any
machine-language subroutines are being loaded from the disk into
memory so the amount of information should be carefully matched
with the time interval required for the loading operation.   As
soon as the BASIC program is loaded it starts and presents the
CRT with its own text.

During the operation of any BASIC program it is possible
for the operator to regain control of the computer by pressing a
RESET button or a CTRL/C combination.   The CRT responds with a
prompting cursor on the bottom line.   At this point the operator

may restart the BASIC program now in memory by simply typing in
RUN and terminating by pressing a RETURN key. Or,
alternatively, another program on the disk may be run by
entering RUN NAME, press RETURN. This will call in the disk
directory (or catalog) and if it contains a program called NAME
it will be loaded and executed.

A student who wishes to restart from the menu
presentation may do so by turning the power off and then on
again. Also it is possible to run the menu-containing program
by name. The author uses the name START for the first program
on the disk, often called the HELLO routine in some circles. In
addition there are a number of short identical programs which do
nothing more than load and run START. These programs are given
names such as MENU, GO, RESTART, SIMULATIONS, etc. so that if an
operator enters a RUN followed by any of these names the called
program will eventually branch to the same menu that is seen for
the power-on situation.

┌─────────────────────┐
│ PROGRAMMING         │
└─────────────────────┘

In many of the chapters there are casual references to
programming techniques which improve the effectiveness and
reliability of the simulation exercises. The following sections
collect these together for emphasis of their importance.

WAITING

During the time that the computer is loading a program
from disk or doing computations it is important to have some
message being displayed on the screen in order to hold
attention. For example, in one version of the Hodgkin-Huxley
simulation there is a period of about 30 seconds at the start of
the program in which the rate constants are evaluated at 1
millivolt increments and stored in a large array. During this
time it is helpful to have the CRT displaying text which
describes to the students what they will be doing during the
exercise, or even explaining that the delay now saves time
later.

One should keep in mind that once an array is
initialized with a set of values many forms of BASIC may wipe
this out on successive executions of a RUN command from the
operator. Similarly after the first simulation has been
finished the program must branch, not to the lowest line number,
but to one after those which fill the arrays. If an operator
should interrupt a running program, as by pressing the RESET
button or CTRL/C combination, entering a GOTO XXX command from

the keyboard will not clear  the    arrays    as    would    a    RUN   XXX
command.

A device to make the waiting time seem to go    faster    is
to  have a count-down clock display how many more seconds remain
until the next step in the exercise.  This can  be    synchronized
with  the   index of the FOR...NEXT loop that is operating during
the delaying operation.

When  the  display of instructions is not locked to some
essential computation or disk operation it is more effective    to
have  the CRT text terminated by having the operator press a key
rather than using a FOR...NEXT loop of finite duration.    If    the
student  has  run the exercise previously or is familar with how
to enter data the instruction text can be skipped over  rapidly.
The  GET  A$  in  some  versions  of  BASIC  waits  for a single
character and does not expect a RETURN key  to  terminate  the
input.    On  the other hand there may be situations where there
are benefits to having the program list  the  objectives  of  an
exercise  one  at  a  time  to be certain that full attention is
given to each.  The computer  language  PILOT  is  designed  for
programming  ease  for  operations  of  this  kind but  is  not
particularly useful in mathematical simulations.


PARAMETER INPUT

There are many opportunities  for  programming  operator
conveniences at the interactive point where the parameters for a
given simulation are being entered.  Default values, chosen  for
normal  conditions of the model, expedite operations by allowing
the parameter to be set by simply pressing the RETURN key.    In
some  versions  of  BASIC  such a response to an INPUT statement
leaves the parameter set to the last assigned value.  In others,
such  a response will give an error message.  In the latter case
if the requested variable is a text string, such as A$, a simple
RETURN response sets the string to a blank.  An IF statement can
then use the VAL(A$) function to assign a numerical value if the
string A$ is not a blank; otherwise, the previously set value is
retained.

In  many instances the numerical value of a parameter in
a model has little meaning in itself but  rather  serves  as  an
index  of  the  sensitivity  of  a process.  For example, in the
simulation  of  the  glucose-insulin  interaction  a  point  of
interest is the amount of insulin released by the pancreas for a
given plasma  glucose  concentration.    Rather  than  put  this
measure  of  sensitivity  into  absolute  units  it is much more
effective to have the INPUT statement ask for a  value  relative
to  normal.    The  program  can  then do the conversion of this
normalized value to the proper absolute values  required  for  a
solution of the model.

A polished simulation program will check each parameter for unreasonable values and give appropriate error messages. For example, a single IF statement can detect negative concentrations and direct the operator to repeat the entry. This "fool-proofing" is a tedious chore but an important one for the successful application of simulation by people with only casual interest in the material.


## CRT DISPLAYS

A rapid, accurate tracing of a function on labeled axes is a powerful aid for anyone lecturing about quantitative and dynamic phenomena. The finite size of the CRT screen and the resolution of the characters and drawings require careful attention to the compromises between presenting adequate information without cluttering it with too much detail. This is an artist endeavor not a science.

When mutiple tracings are to be superimposed on the same axes, such as the sodium and potassium conductances during an action potential, assigning different colors to each tracing is a great help. In lieu of this an individual tracing can be identified as a dashed curve by having it displayed on alternate values of the abscissa. However this is not effective if the variable selected is changing rapidly. Thus during the action potential the potassium conductance is the more desirable variable to be plotted as an interrupted tracing.

When CRT space permits it is helpful to retain the key parameters of the model being simulated so that the student does not forget the purpose of the exercise. Examples are the parameters of stimuli for an action potential, pancreatic sensitiviites for the glucose tolerance test, and the angle of deviation of the electrical axis of the heart for a vectorcardiogram.


## ANOTHER APPROACH

Most of the simulation exercises in this book have given the student an opportunity to select any arbitrary value of the parameters from a very wide range of reasonable values for a given model. This provides maximum flexibility in probing the process under study but the extent of the choices may be overwhelming for the casual student. Dr. Ramon Gonzalez, Jr. of Loma Linda University uses microcomputers for teaching physiology and provides alternative programs designed for such situations. This approach should be of general interest.

The general idea is to preselect certain combinations of model parameters as illustrating specific properties of the

physiological system under study.  Once the exercise is selected
from a menu presentation, as in Figure  14.1,  successive  menus
present  specific  alternative  disturbances  to  the  simulated
system.  This narrows the range of choice of such parameters  as
a  nerve  stimulus  amplitude and duration to those appropriate,
for example, for  subthreshold,  threshold,  and  suprathreshold
responses.   An  entirely  different program may be called with
options presented to demonstrate another property, such  as  the
refractory period of the nerve axon.

        Besides focusing student attention upon meaningful input
values  this  approach  can  speed  up  simulations  which might
ordinarily require numerous time-consuming iterations.   Because
of the limited range of combinations it may be possible to store
all of the possible responses  and  have  the  menu  select  the
appropriate  one.   This  is  analogous to viewing figures in a
textbook, but the  process  of  selection  by  the  student  and
microcomputer  viewing makes the process an active one which may
have a lasting effect.

        To  simplify the interaction between the student and the
computer it is possible to replace the console keyboard with  an
input  device  which has a limited number of possible responses.
A simple keypad with only 10 digits, termination key, and  reset
button  is  one  approach.    Dr. Gonzalez uses a "light pen", a
photoelectric detector which  the  student  places  on  the  CRT
screen  opposite  the  selected  option  in  a  menu.   Once the
selection is made the software does a variety of things, such as
read  an  exercise  from  disk into memory or apply a new set of
input parameters to a chosen model.  In this context the student
need  see  and  interact only with what is on the CRT screen and
that display can be made as simple or complex as the  instructor
may  wish.   The microcomputer can be out of sight and relegated
to a minor role as far as the student is concerned.

        This  alternative  method  of  setting  up  a simulation
exercise is presented as the final page of this book because  it
illustrates  that microcomputers are indeed personal possessions
under the control of individual instructors.  The programming in
BASIC is straight-forward enough that teachers of physiology can
mold their microcomputers' potential to  suit  their  own  local
teaching  approach.   The development of the new technology is a
creative experience for the instructor whose enthusiasm  carries
over to the students involved.

INDEX

Accommodation, 182-183
Accuracy of computation, 189, 217
Action potential
  axon, 6, 48, 157-198
  cardiac, 199-224
Address, 13
Address bus, 10
Afterload, 84, 88
ALTAIR
  S-100 bus, 42, 48, 55, 172
  microcomputer, 24
Am-9511 numerical processor, 36,
    45-47, 192, 220
Analog computers, 4
Anode-break excitation, 182
Apple II, 11, 25, 31, 41, 47, 52,
    125, 174, 216
Applesoft BASIC, 53, 189, 194
Arithmetic Processor Unit (APU), 36,
    45-47, 192, 220
Arterial pulse pressure, 116-128
Assemblers, 34, 193-194
ASCII code, 19, 40
Audio cassette, 20
Autoregressive difference equation,
    145
Autostart ROM, 53, 226
Axon action potential, 6, 48,
    157-198

BASIC, 35, 53,
BASIC programs
  axon action potential, 159-169
  cardiac action potential, 201-208
  cardiovascular mechanics, 85-90
  insulin-glucose interaction, 73-76
  pulse pressure, 121-125
  sequential compartments, 61-64
  vectorcardiogram, 133-137
  waveform distortion, 150-151
Beeler-Reuter model, 199-224

Bit, 13
Bloodflow, 89, 124
Blood pressure
  mean, 89
  pulse, 116
  waveform, 143
Blood volume, 87, 104
Bus, 10, 24, 53
Byte, 13

Calcium
  current, 203, 210, 213
  intracellular, 201, 203
Capacitance, membrane, 167
Cardiovascular models, 2, 5, 83, 116
Cardiac output, 84, 89, 103, 119
Cathode ray tube (CRT), 17-20,
    40-44, 230
Clock, 10, 12
Compartmental kinetics, 57
Computer-aided-instruction (CAI), 6
Computers
  analog, 4
  digital, 5
  microcomputers, 1, 6, 9, 50-56
  time-shared, 6
Compiler, 37, 48
Compliance, vascular, 87, 104
Computation
  accuracy, 189, 217
  speed, 188, 219
Computed responses of models
  axon action potential, 177-186
  cardiac action potential, 208-214
  cardiovascular mechanics, 101-111
  compartmental kinetics, 59-61
  glucose tolerance test, 76-78
  pulse pressure, 118-121
  vectorcardiography, 131-133
  waveform distortion, 141-144
Conductance, membrane, 161, 164, 179

Contractility, cardiac, 87, 101
CP/M, 22, 32-34, 55
Currents
    constant stimulus, 184, 214
    potassium, 161-164, 203, 213
    slow, 200, 203, 210, 213
    sodium, 161-164, 203, 211, 214
Data bus, 10, 14
Deconvolution, 148
Deviation of electrical axis, 132
Diabetes, 70
Difference equation, 145
Differential equations, 4, 8, 63,
    109, 116, 145, 165, 207
Digital computers, 5
Digital filtering, 145
Disks, 22
Disk operating system (DOS), 30
Dynamic memory, 16


Electrical axis, 132
Electrocardiogram (ECG), 129, 150
Euler integration, 63, 105, 145,
    169, 187, 207, 217
Excitation
    axon, 157-198
    cardiac, 199-224
    properties of, 177-187


Firmware, 53
First-order process, 4, 57, 63, 141,
    145
Floating point
    numbers, 14, 193
    processors, 36, 45-47, 192, 220
Floppy disks, 22, 33, 226
Format, 99, 110, 225
FORTH, 37, 47
FORTRAN, 37, 70, 159, 188


Graphics, 40, 69, 133, 172, 174, 216
Gaussian elimination, 95
Glucose tolerance test, 69-82
Glucose-insulin interation, 70-73


Hard-sector disk format, 22
HCOLOR command, 42, 176
Hexadecimal number, 13

High-resolution graphics, 39
Hodgkin-Huxley model, 3, 158
HPLOT command, 42, 54, 125, 176
Hypertension, 103
Hypertrophy, cardiac 98
Hypoglycemia, 69


Integration,  63, 105, 145, 169,
    187, 217
Inhibition rebound, 182
Initial conditions, 162, 204
Input/output ports, 14, 42, 46
Insulin-glucose interaction, 70-73
Integer
    numbers, 13, 45
    BASIC, 153
Integrated circuits, 11
Inverse filter, 148


Keyboard, 10, 16


Large-scale-integration (LSI) 14, 11
Light pen, 231
Limb leads for ECG, 129
Low-pass filter, 143


Machine language, 34, 192-194
Macrocomputer, 7
Mass storage, 20
Mathematical models, 3
Mechanical models, 2
Membrane currents, 164, 203
Memory
    dynamic, 16
    display buffer, 19
    read-only-memory (ROM), 15
    random-access-memory (RAM), 15
    semiconductor, 14
Memory-mapped I/O, 14, 19
Menu, 54, 226, 231
Microcomputers, 1, 6, 9, 24, 39,
    50-56
    See TRS-80, Apple II, SOL-20
Microprocessors
    6502, 11, 194
    8080/8085, 48
    Z-80, 11, 51

Models
  analog, 4
  arterial pulse pressure, 116-118
  axon action potential, 159-169
  cardiovascular mechanics, 85-94
  cardiac action potential, 201-208
  compartmental kinetics, 58-59
  insulin-glucose interaction, 70-73
  mathematical, 3
  mechanical, 2
  respiration, 2,4,
Modulator, 18
Monitors
  software, 30-32, 53
  video, 10, 18
Motherboard, 24, 53


Numbers
  integer, 13, 153
  floating point, 14, 36, 45-47, 193
  octal, 13
  hexidecimal, 13
  binary, 13
Numerical processors, 36, 45-47,
    192, 220


Octal number, 13
Operating systems, 29, 31
Operation code, 13
Output displays, 42, 46, 96, 170,
    215


Pancreas, 72
Parameter input, 91, 118, 134, 162,
    229
PET microcomputer, 21
PILOT, 37
Pixels, 18
PLATO, 6
Poiseuille's law, 84
Potassium currents, 161-164, 203
Programming, 228


Random-access-memory (RAM), 15
Rate constants, 58, 165, 202
Read-only-memory (ROM), 15, 53
Refractory period, 183
Resistance, vascular, 87, 103, 120

Respiration model, 2, 4
Restoring distorted waveforms,
    147-149
Reverse Polish notation, 38


S-100 bus, 42, 48, 55, 172
Sector of disk, 22
Semiconductor memory, 14
Serial video terminals, 19
Simulation, 7
Sinusoidal input, 142
Slow response, 213
Slow current, 200
Sodium currents
  axon, 161-164
  cardiac, 203, 211
SOL-20 microcomputer, 25, 55
SOLOS operating system, 30
Soft-sector disks, 23
Speed of computation, 188, 219
Stack, 45
Static gain, 145
Stimulus parameters, 164
Steady-state, 91, 101, 166
Student exercises, 225


Tabular displays, 96, 110, 170
Temporal summation, 181
Threaded-code compiler, 37
Threshold to excitation, 178
Time constant, 59, 144-145
Transient solutions, 105
Transistor-transistor-logic (TTL),
    12
TRS-80 microcomputer, 11, 25, 31,
    41, 46, 51, 171
Turnkey systems, 226
TV raster, 17, 43


Vectorcardiography, 129
Venous return curves, 84, 100
Ventricular function curves, 84, 100
Video monitors, 43
Voltage clamp, 186


Waveform distortion, 140
Windkessel model, 84, 116
Word, defined, 12